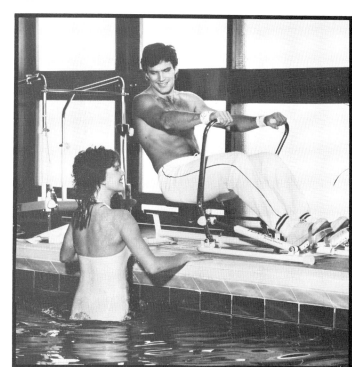

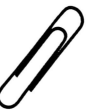

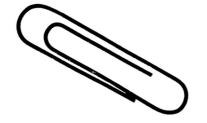

HomeWork-out

By Richard Edel

wcb
Wm. C. Brown Publishers
Dubuque, Iowa

Library of Congress Catalog Number 84–73458

ISBN 0-697-00711-1

Printed in the United States of America
10 9 8 7 6 5 4 3 2 1

Acknowledgements

HomeWork-out is based on extensive research from a variety of information sources, including manufacturers, physiologists, doctors, dieticians, designers, engineers, reference books, textbooks, and others. But it would not have been possible without the tireless help of two individuals: Geoffrey Shives, art director and designer, and Patrick Kirk, trade editor for Wm. C. Brown Co. Publishers. To both of these individuals, I am indebted and grateful.

Special credit also goes to Tom Eitter, Ph.D., who reviewed the book and provided technical advice, and to the manufacturers of home fitness equipment, who provided information, photography, and unlimited assistance in the preparation of the manuscript.

Portions of *HomeWork-out* are adapted from the following publications: Self-assessment tests from *Physical Fitness,* by Marilyn Snyder Halper, M.P.H., and Ira Neiger. Copyright 1980 by Preventive Medicine Institute/Strang Clinic. Reprinted by permission of Holt, Rinehart and Winston, Publishers.

The section and illustrations of stretching exercises are adapted from *Physical Activity . . . For Fitness and Health,* 1981, reprinted with permission of the American Medical Association.

The section dealing with heart rates and workload capacities is adapted from *Physical Fitness: How To Plan For It, Reach Your Goal and Measure Your Progress,* with permission of Vitamaster, Div. Allegheny Int'l Exercise Co. Additional acknowledgement goes to Blair D. Erb, M.D., who assisted and contributed to preparation of the Vitamaster booklet.

The section on "Eating right" was adapted with permission from four publications of the American Medical Association: *Your Age & Your Diet,* 1983; *Vitamin-Mineral Supplements and Physical Activity . . . For Fitness and Health,* 1981; Their Correct Use, 1981; *Sodium And Your Health,* no date.

I would also like to thank Christopher Colletti for preparation of chart materials, and assistance in graphic design; Cecelia Reed, for suggestions on editorial development and content; James Enterprises for color separations; and the many others who have been generous with their time, and were helpful in many ways.

Richard Edel

Cover models: Cathy Nale and Steve Karegeannes

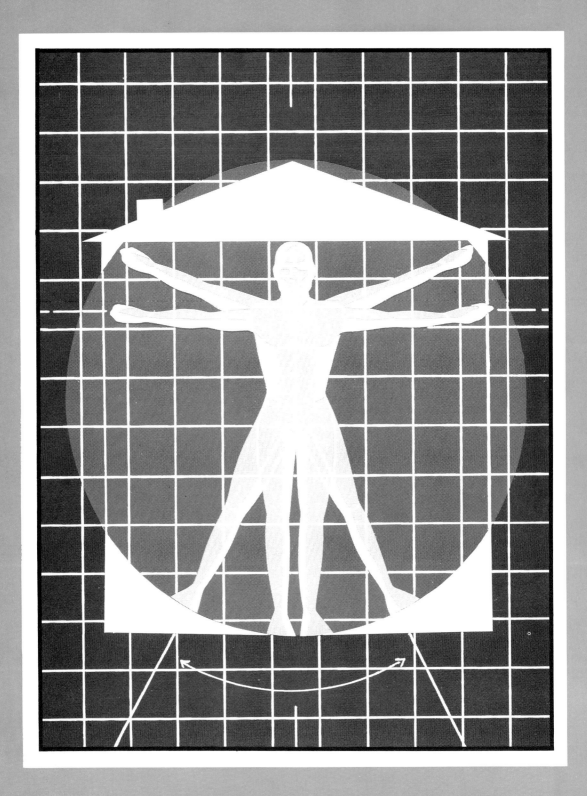

Contents

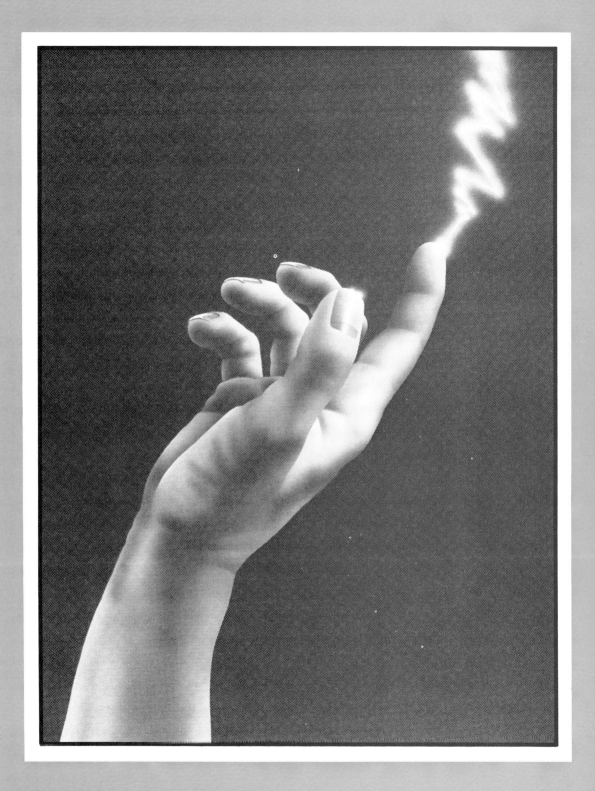

Choices

Making the grade

You made a secret promise at some time in your life to improve your body. Everyone does. Perhaps your goal was to lose weight, or maybe you decided to put on some muscle. But for one reason or another, something always got in the way. Your promise was put off until tomorrow.

Your physical condition isn't likely to improve unless you make an important lifestyle choice: to start an exercise program. It's a difficult choice, but a good one. A few hours each week for home fitness can make you healthier, better looking, and happier.

Use *HomeWork-out* as your guide to selecting the right home fitness equipment and creating an exercise plan designed just for you. It's a workbook for your life.

HomeWork-out can help you to keep that promise you made long ago. You *can* make the grade.

Back to school

Whether you realize it or not, you are continually teaching your body (and mind) to adjust to your lifestyle at work and at home. *HomeWork-out* is a guide to re-educating your body to a new life of vigor and activity. It offers lessons in endurance, strength, and flexibility, based on a foundation of good nutrition.

HomeWork-out is your guide to the best home gym equipment at prices you can afford. And it describes how to create a personalized fitness program tailor made to your needs and goals.

Think back to the trim, firm body you had (or would like to have had) in high school or college. It can still be yours.

With *HomeWork-out,* you will look better

and, most importantly, you will *feel better,* about both yourself and your body.

Why home fitness?

You may want to improve your lifestyle by starting a fitness program, but there may be reasons why you cannot attend an exercise class or join a health club. In many cases, time is short or daily pressures conflict with the open hours. You may feel embarrassed working out alongside well developed bodybuilders. Or you may need time to lose a few pounds and tone up before getting serious.

Whatever your reasons, the best place to begin exercising is in the home, whether or not you also take an exercise class, swim, bicycle, or run. Why? Because it is convenient and because home exercise gets results. You have fewer excuses to skip a workout. A home gym is there during bad weather, before and after work, and when you have little time to spare.

Time, by the way, is a key factor in working out at home. Whereas a trip to the gym might occupy a day or an evening, exercising at home can give you the same results in a fraction of the time.

Cost is another good reason for exercising at home. A huge variety of quality home equipment is now available at affordable prices. Commercial gymnasiums no longer have a monopoly on the best products. (Most home exercise equipment shown in this book was not available until recently.)

You can buy single or multi-station home

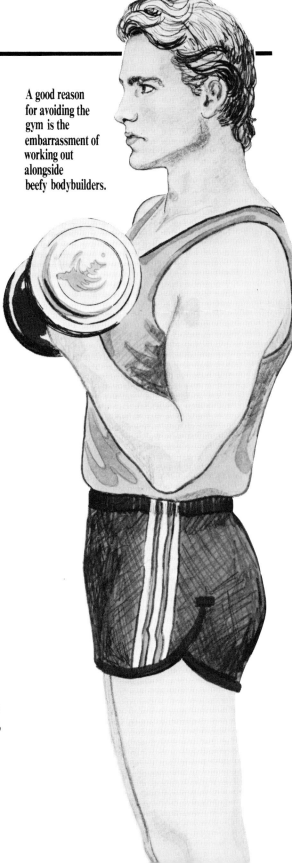

A good reason for avoiding the gym is the embarrassment of working out alongside beefy bodybuilders.

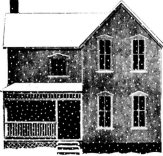

A home gym is there during bad weather, before and after work and when you have little time to spare.

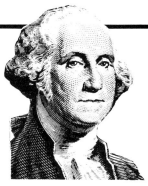

A variety of home fitness equipment is now available at affordable prices.

exercise machines at prices on par or less than the cost of joining a gym.

But the best reason for home fitness is you. It gives you the means to achieve better weight control, increased strength and endurance, improved coordination and general appearance. And it gives you a good feeling about yourself.

Mind, body and spirit, home fitness is tailor-made for you and your good health.

Cramming

Enthusiasm will take you far in your new home fitness routine, but you cannot undo years of physical neglect in a short time. Moderation is urged; overexertion is the main reason that many quickly abandon a newly begun exercise routine.

Getting into shape at home does not mean radically altering your daily habits. All that is required for home exercise is a few minutes in

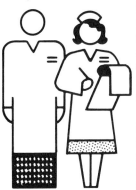

the morning, afternoon or evening a few days each week for a workout. Start slowly and work progressively towards more difficult exercises.

Consult a physician before engaging in strenuous exercise, especially if you are overweight, on medication, or have been inactive for a long period of time. Even if you are in great

Even if you are in great shape, a periodic check-up is advised by doctors.

shape, a periodic check-up is advised by doctors.

As your physical condition improves, you will notice an enhancement in the quality of the things you enjoy. Food, drink, relaxation, work, sex: all are more pleasurable if you are active and feel alive. This is true for men and women, young and old.

Report cards

Periodically in *HomeWork-out,* you will be tested on your performance. But don't worry, a lower than average test result is not an indication of failure, but a guide to isolate areas where you may need additional work.

Start by giving yourself an "A" for picking up this book: you have the desire to get into shape. Now let's see if you have the motivation. Let's get started!

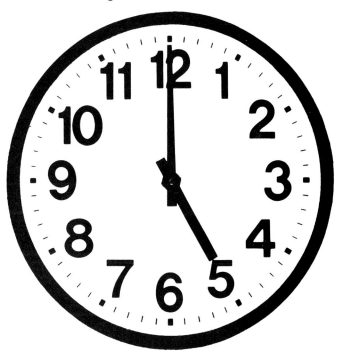

Time and how much of it you save, is a good reason to start a home fitness program.

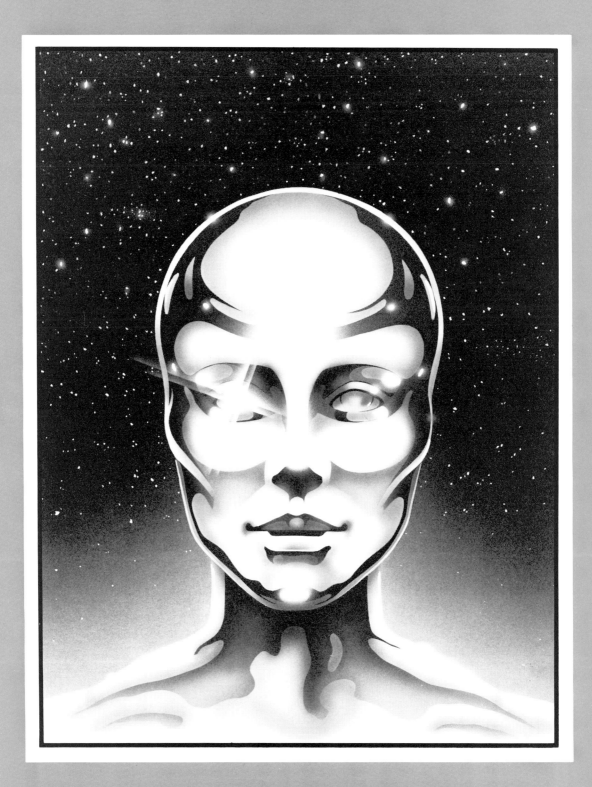

Lifestyle

Taking inventory

Before you rush out to buy home fitness equipment and embark on an exercise program, take a moment to rediscover your body. Conduct a personal inventory of every curve and line, forgetting for the time being how you would eventually like to appear.

Stand unclothed in front of a full-length mirror and give yourself a thorough visual examination. Try to avoid being too critical; pretend, for the moment, that you are looking at yourself for the first time. At this stage, it is

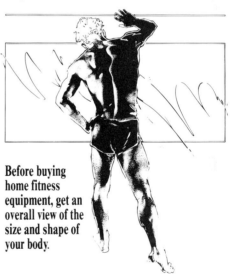

Before buying home fitness equipment, get an overall view of the size and shape of your body.

important to remain objective so that you can set attainable goals in an exercise program.

It may help you to begin your examination with the general and work to the specific. First, get an overall view of the size and shape of your body, turning so that you can see yourself from different angles. Is your frame stocky, average, or lean? How tall are you in relation to your weight? Are you carrying a few extra pounds? How broad are your shoulders and hips? Are they in proportion to your height? Perhaps you could benefit by gaining a few pounds in the right places while losing a few in others.

Next, concentrate on the specifics. Is your neck long and shapely, short and thick, or is it nondescript? How about your shoulders? Are they muscular, lean, or shapeless? Are your arms and legs fleshy, shapely, or linear? Is your chest or bosom deep and full or narrow and thin? Does your abdomen seem toned or does it bulge? Is your waistline under control?

Isolate every part of your body and give it an objective appraisal, making mental notes about what, in general and in particular, you would like to improve.

Pinch test

As a second phase of your self-examination, give yourself a few well-placed squeezes, for example, on your arms, legs, waistline, buttocks and abdomen. How does your body feel? Is it squeezably soft or pleasantly firm?

If your flesh feels soft and spongy, you probably lead a relatively sedentary lifestyle. Flesh, which is made up mostly of fat and muscle tissue, generally will feel doughy and soft unless you exercise regularly. Toned muscles are springy and firm to the touch. They don't droop, roll, or hang.

No body's perfect

Ever wonder why some people tend to gain or lose weight more easily than others? Or why some tone up quickly with seemingly little effort while others take much longer? The reason is that your body responds at its own pace to diet and exercise. In addition, body type, age, sex, and physical condition all have varying effects on your ability to lose or gain weight and on how quickly you are able to build or tone muscles. You can be a knockout at fifty or a washout at thirty, depending on your natural traits and on what you do (or don't do) to enhance them. No body is perfect. You have to work on it.

Body basics

In general, there are three body types: endomorphic (stocky build), mesomorphic (average build), and ectomorphic (lean build). You may fit easily into one category, or, like most people, your body may be a combination of all three body types. Regardless, it is helpful for the moment to decide approximately where you belong.

Stocky If your body type is stocky, or endomorphic, you tend to have a greater fat body weight composition. Because of your thicker limbs and heavier build, as an endomorph, you have to work extra hard at eating right and shaping your physique. But, the results of regular hard workouts may surprise and delight you.

Average If you are a mesomorph, your body is characterized mostly by its greater muscle weight composition. Mesomorphs tend to readily show muscular definition with exercise. You are fortunate genetically. This body type is one that closely matches today's standard of beauty, according to the characteristics that advertisers look for in male and female models. However, before you decide that, as a mesomorph, you don't really need exercise after all, think how much better you would look if you were toned up and trimmed down.

And don't forget the importance of cardiovascular conditioning in keeping your health and your shape. You have been given the best raw physical material. What you do with it is up to you.

Lean The ectomorphic body tends to have the least body fat and muscle. The predominant characteristic is a slight build with linear and narrow features. Arms and legs generally are long and slender and less shapely than endomorphic and mesomorphic body types.

The expression "you can never be too rich or too thin" notwithstanding, you can benefit greatly from exercise even with an extremely ectomorphic body. Put simply, the benefit is that toned muscle shows more

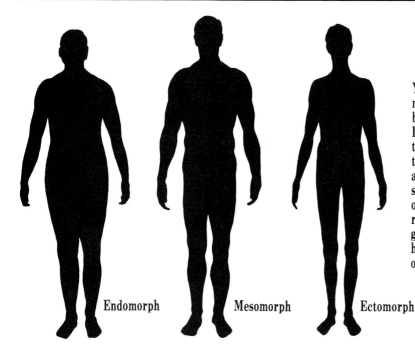

Your body is the raw material that is sculpted by an exercise program. In general, there are three extremes of body type, shown at the left, although most people show traits of more than one type. No matter what raw material you were given, home exercise can help you make the most of it.

Endomorph   Mesomorph   Ectomorph

definition than untoned, which means exercise can add shape to your body. Exercise and proper diet can bring out the rich characteristics inherent in a lean frame.

Starting out

You might have the best intentions of taking positive action with your life, but may be hesitant about how much you can do or where to begin. Here are a few things to consider.

Medical examination: If you haven't had a complete physical recently, get one before you begin any strenuous home exercise. Tell your doctor exactly what you plan to do, including the type of exercise you are considering, anticipated changes in diet or eating habits, and anything else you can think of. Specifically ask if the doctor would recommend any limits on exercise. Even the best, most highly trained athletes visit with their doctors frequently. Those who don't court potential disaster.

Your age: It is a common misbelief that aging places limitations on vigorous physical activity. The truth is that unless there is an actual physical problem, it usually is the individual who determines the limits. The newspapers are full of stories about marathon runners who began training in their sixties and seventies, and about elderly men and women who are top-notch athletes in their sports and classes.

Extensive research at major universities shows that men and women who are physically active in middle age are more likely to age successfully than those who are sedentary. "Success," in this case, means the ability to function physically and the capacity to lead a happy, fulfilling life. These people do not necessarily lead longer lives, but rather lives that are busier and more free of the usual problems of aging.

There is growing evidence that a healthy, active lifestyle also plays an important role in forestalling the onset of certain degenerative diseases. These are conditions that occur as a result of heredity and aging. For example, regular, sustained physical activity reduces the symptoms of arthritis and keeps them at bay longer.

Even if you already have stiff joints, fallen arches, an expanding girth, and a lifestyle that focuses more on television than home fitness, with an intelligent plan, it is never too late to change. Don't follow the example of W.C. Fields, who claimed that when he felt the urge to exercise, he would lie down until it passed.

Think of aging as a strong motivation for working to improve your lifestyle.

Sexuality: Many women worry that, with regular exercise, they will become as muscular as men. Nothing could be farther from the

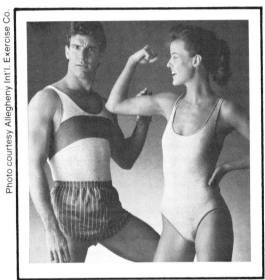

It is a mistaken notion that, with regular exercise, a woman would become as muscular as a man.

truth. Because a woman has lower levels of hormones that encourage muscle-building, it is virtually impossible for her to achieve the same level of muscularity as a man. Generally, home exercise will cause a woman to lose body fat and tone muscles in selected areas. Because a woman normally carries a greater percentage of body fat than a man, the result will be a more rounded shapeliness.

A man, on the other hand, may set optimistic goals of building muscle or endurance and attempt to start right off with strenuous home exercise. While he may achieve great results, he also may begin to

experience discomfort from sore, stiff muscles and tendons. Male musculature, by nature, is not as flexible as that of a female, and requires more time for stretching and limbering up.

In general, for both men and women, it is best to begin a program of exercise upon which you feel you can most comfortably build. If you have not regularly engaged in strenuous exercise in the recent past, start slowly and work toward progressively more difficult routines.

It is also wise to be realistic about your physique, in terms of its assets and liabilities. If you have wide hips and narrow shoulders, no amount of exercise can reverse the order. However, you could surprise yourself by how good your body would look if you allowed it to reach its full potential.

Vital signs

Home fitness involves the development of all aspects of your physical potential. It has three basic components: flexibility, muscle conditioning and aerobic conditioning. While the three categories overlap somewhat, it may help to look first at each individually and then show how they can work together in a unified home fitness plan.

Flexibility: Unless you maintain a physically active lifestyle, your muscles, ligaments, and tendons generally shorten and stiffen as you age. Over time, this limits your ability to move, bend, and use your body. You also become more susceptible to injury because your muscles are more easily stressed to their limits.

Regular stretching helps muscles, tendons, and ligaments to remain long and supple. A full range of stretching exercises is presented in the back of this book along with information about how your body changes with exercise.

Muscle conditioning: Basically, this means developing and strengthening muscles through resistance training. Lifting weights is the most efficient method of resistance

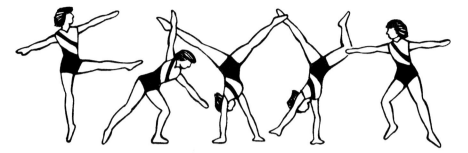

Running, walking, swimming, bicycling, and other such activities, all are excellent ways of improving aerobic fitness.

training. When you lift weights, gravity opposes your muscles and they gradually grow, adapting to greater and greater resistance.

Home fitness machines duplicate the resistance of gravity in many clever ways. Many, in fact, incorporate variable weight stacks in their designs. As your muscles grow stronger, you periodically increase the resistance, or weight, and continue to progress.

Home fitness makes it easy and convenient to reap the benefits of weight lifting without the mess and trouble of free weights.

Aerobic conditioning: Aerobic means ''living in the presence of oxygen.'' Aerobic conditioning means developing your *cardiovascular endurance,* or your body's ability to supply oxygen to your muscles through the combined effort of the heart, lungs, and circulatory system.

Improving your aerobic conditioning requires continuous exercise at gradually increasing time intervals. Running, walking, swimming, sculling, bicycling, and other such activities all are excellent means of improving aerobic fitness. Even better, in many instances, is the use of home fitness machines designed to duplicate the action and results of these activities.

Treadmills, exercise bicycles, rowing machines, and other devices not only give you the same returns for your effort, they can be set up in the comfort of your own home. No more trips to the park in the rain, or weaving through busy traffic on foot or bicycle to get your daily workout.

Looking good—feeling better

Your age, sex, and emotional and physical conditions are important factors in planning and implementing a home exercise program. These same factors should be taken into account when you periodically evaluate your progress. The most important consideration, however, is your lifestyle. Is it working for you?

Lifestyle with style

The term *lifestyle* encompasses everything you *do* with your life as opposed to facts *about* your life, such as how old you are. Is your lifestyle an active or sedate one? Do you spend a lot of time engaged in leisure pursuits or do you participate in vigorous activities? What do you do in the course of a normal day at work or at home? Do you drink or smoke?

Never mind the occasional night out that ends early the next day, or the holiday food orgy. Think about your lifestyle in terms of how you have lived over the past few years, not days.

Your lifestyle has far-reaching effects on the business, social and private aspects of your life. Think how much better your relationships and activities could be if your lifestyle gave you the vitality to enjoy them to the fullest.

Getting physical

A vital component of a lifestyle with style is regular physical activity. And the best way to accommodate it in your busy schedule is with a home gym.

You think, feel, and operate better when your body is conditioned. You are more mentally alert, better able to relax and sleep, and are less susceptible to physical and emotional stress. You also are more able to bounce back from minor injuries, aches, and pains when you are in shape.

Experts say that the onset of many health problems can be delayed or their effects minimized by a lifestyle that incorporates regular exercise. To a greater or lesser degree, you can take steps through home exercise to reduce the risk of many problems, such as obesity, heart attack, smoking-related diseases, high blood pressure, chronic fatigue, depression, and anxiety.

Obviously, regular exercise is not the only way to reduce the risk of disease and improving your business and personal life. But frequent exercise has a highly positive effect on your physical and mental well-being.

Setting goals

There is more to total home fitness than the three physical components—flexibility, muscle conditioning, and aerobic conditioning—that were described in this section. The most

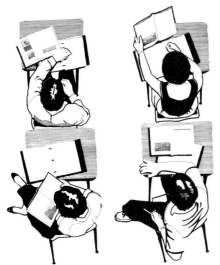

important factors are in your mind. What do you hope to gain from a home exercise program? How motivated are you to make it work for you?

This chapter is designed to help you decide for yourself which goals are most important to you, how motivated you really are, and what degree of success you might expect from a home fitness program. Once you identify what motivates you to exercise, designing your routine and selecting the proper equipment is easy. The hard part is doing it.

Self-assessment

There are three self-assessments in this chapter. Test 1 will help you to determine your attitude toward exercise. Test 2 will help you to assess your present level of physical activity. Test 3 will help you to clarify your specific goals for home fitness.

Profile record

Concluding the chapter is a "profile record," where you will be asked to record the results of the three self-assessment activities. Your profile record will help you to establish your goals for home exercise in order of priority. It would be wise to refer to this record often in designing your home fitness program. In this way, the conditioning program and fitness equipment that you select will reflect *your* goals—not those, for example, of some celebrity-turned-exercise-guru.

Setting specific and realistic goals for yourself (and who is more qualified for this than you?) is the first step in developing a successful home fitness program. It is the yardstick against which you measure your progress over time.

One general goal that you can set right now is to include regular home exercise as a part of your everyday life. Long after you reach those early, specific goals of losing weight or toning up, a program of regular exercise will help you to remain in peak condition.

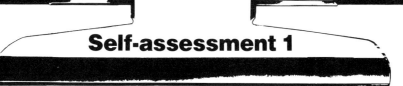

Self-assessment 1

What is your attitude toward exercise ?

After reading each statement, circle the number that most accurately indicates how you feel. For example, in question "a," if you strongly agree, circle "1," if you agree, circle "2," and so on. Be sure to answer every question.

		Strongly agree	Agree	Disagree	Strongly disagree
a	Basically I am a sedentary (inactive) person.	1	2	3	4
b	Exercise is enjoyable.	4	3	2	1
c	When I was a child, my family encouraged me to exercise.	4	3	2	1
d	Exercise is boring.	1	2	3	4
e	The ability to master a fitness program would be an exciting challenge to me.	4	3	2	1
f	I avoid physical activity.	1	2	3	4
g	I have an increased sense of well-being after I exercise vigorously.	4	3	2	1
h	I usually find excuses not to exercise.	1	2	3	4
i	Maintaining a physical fitness program would show that I have willpower.	4	3	2	1
j	Looking good is very important to me.	4	3	2	1
k	Physically fit people always look better.	4	3	2	1
l	I don't like looking unfit.	4	3	2	1

Self-assessment tests from *Physical Fitness*, by Marilyn Snyder Halper, M.P.H. and Ira Neiger. Copyright 1980 by Preventive Medicine Institute/Strang Clinic. Reprinted by permission of Holt, Rinehart and Winston, Publishers.

How to score

Enter the numbers you have circled in response to the statements in Self-Assessment 1 in the appropriate spaces below. Write the number you circled for statement "a" over line "a," the number for statement "b" over line "b," and so on. Add the scores across and record the total. For example, the sum of your scores over lines "a," "c," and "f" gives your total score for "Image."

After you have added up your scores, read "How to Interpret Your Scores" and enter your scores on the "Profile Record," on page 17.

___ a + ___ c + ___ f = ___ IMAGE

___ b + ___ d + ___ g = ___ ENJOYMENT

___ j + ___ k + ___ l = ___ APPEARANCE

___ e + ___ h + ___ i = ___ DISCIPLINE

How to interpret your scores

Scores can vary from three to twelve. A score of nine or above is high. A score of six or under is low. A score of seven or eight is average.

Image

If you scored nine or above on "Image," you probably think of yourself as a fairly active person.

If you want to be as slender as a ballerina, or as burly as a bodybuilder, you have to share their *attitudes* toward diet and exercise.

Applying this positive image toward your home exercise program will contribute to your success.

If you scored six or below, you may be hampered by a negative image of yourself. A sedentary image is often inherited from one's family. A regular home fitness program will help you to improve that image.

Enjoyment

If you scored nine or above, you already enjoy exercise. This ability will help you maintain a regular long-term home fitness program.

If you scored six or below you probably do not enjoy exercising. Remember: you can take steps to make home exercise more pleasant. Try working out with a friend, exercising to music, or finding a more pleasant location.

Appearance

If you scored nine or above, your appearance is quite important to you. Your positive attitude in regard to your appearance will help you to succeed in establishing a home exercise program.

If you scored six or below, appearance is not your most important motivation for fitness. But keep in mind that a fit figure is attractive at any age.

Discipline

If you scored nine or above, it is important to you to be in control of your life. This attitude will serve as an effective tool in helping you succeed with a regular home fitness program.

If you scored six or below, making use of record-keeping charts should be encouraging, and the process itself should aid you in learning to control your daily patterns and habits.

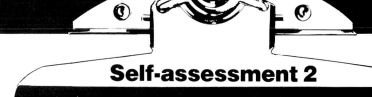

Self-assessment 2

What is your present level of physical activity?

Read each statement and circle the number that most accurately describes how you feel. For example, in question "a," if you always feel that way, circle "4," if you often do, circle "3," and so on. Be sure to answer every question.

	Always	Often	Sometimes	Never
a I walk rather than ride whenever possible.	4	3	2	1
b I exercise more than once a week.	4	3	2	1
c I don't have enough time to exercise.	1	2	3	4
d I use stairs rather than elevators or escalators.	4	3	2	1
e I have a formal exercise plan that I follow.	4	3	2	1
f I find time every day to do something active.	4	3	2	1
g Most of my workday is spent sitting behind a desk.	1	2	3	4
h I participate in some sport (tennis, dancing, jogging, swimming) at least once a week.	4	3	2	1

How to score

Enter the numbers you have circled in response to the statements in Self-Assessment 2 in the appropriate spaces below. Write the number you circled for statement "a" over line "a," the number for statement "b" over line "b," and so on. Add the scores across and record the total. For example, the sum of your scores over lines "b," "c," "e," and "h" gives your total score for "Exercise."

After you have added up your scores, read "How to Interpret Your Scores," and enter your scores on the "Profile Record" on page 17.

__b + __c + __e + __h = __EXERCISE

__a + __d + __f + __g = __ACTIVITY

How to interpret your scores

Scores can vary from four to sixteen. A score of twelve or above is high. A score of eight or under is low. A score of nine to eleven is average.

Exercise

If you scored twelve or above, you already exercise fairly regularly and are well on your way to a successful home fitness program. You may have to increase your current level of exercise only slightly. Look carefully at your goals and remodel your present program to fit them.

If you scored eight or below, you are probably not exercising enough. Pay close attention to the exercises and stretches suggested in this book and to those suggested by the makers of home fitness equipment. They take only a modest amount of time, and if you stick with them, you will be amazed at how much they can do for you.

Activity

If you scored twelve or above, you lead a fairly active life. You may want to increase the amount of your daily activity and include a regular exercise program. Because you are already active, you are on the right track.

If you scored eight or below, you are probably an inactive person. You do not tend to think of active ways to do everyday things. Increasing the number of times you walk, climb stairs, and move from place to place each day can improve your body function and prepare you for an exercise program.

Composite score

Add your total exercise score and your total activity score to compute your composite score. Your composite score will help you to select the appropriate level of exercise at which to begin. Enter your total activity score on your "Profile Record," page 17.

How to score

Enter the numbers you have circled in response to the statements in Self-

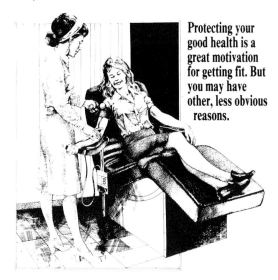

Protecting your good health is a great motivation for getting fit. But you may have other, less obvious reasons.

Self-assessment 3

Why do you want to be physically fit?

The following are reasons people frequently give to explain why they want to be physically fit and what they hope to gain from a fitness program. Circle the number that best describes your attitude. For example, if you think reason "a" is extremely important. circle "4," if you think it is fairly important, circle "3," and so on. Be sure to answer every question.

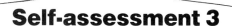

		Extremely Important	Fairly Important	Not very Important	Unimportant
a	To protect myself from heart problems.	4	3	2	1
b	To have more energy.	4	3	2	1
c	To increase my work efficiency.	4	3	2	1
d	To relieve my feelings of tiredness.	4	3	2	1
e	To relieve tension.	4	3	2	1
f	To trim my waist.	4	3	2	1
g	To streamline my body.	4	3	2	1
h	To help me sleep better.	4	3	2	1
i	To relieve stress.	4	3	2	1
j	To increase my wind capacity.	4	3	2	1
k	To eliminate bulges.	4	3	2	1
l	To tighten sagging muscles.	4	3	2	1
m	To lose weight.	4	3	2	1
n	To lower my blood pressure.	4	3	2	1
o	To protect myself from injury and accidents.	4	3	2	1

Assessment 3 in the appropriate spaces below. Write the number you circled for statement "a" over line "a," the number for statement "b" over line "b," and so on. Add the scores across and record the total. For example, the sum of your scores over lines "a," "j," and "n" gives your total score for "Heart Rate and Respiratory Reserve."

After you have added up your scores, read "How to Interpret Your Scores" and enter your scores on the "Profile Record" on page 17.

___a +___ j +___n = ___ HEART RATE AND RESPIRATORY RESERVE

___e +___ h +___j = ___ STRESS AND TENSION RELIEF

___b +___c +___d = ___ ENERGY

___g +___ l +___c = ___ MUSCLE TONE AND GENERAL CONDITIONING

___f +___k +___m = ___ FAT REDUCTION

How to interpret your scores

A score of nine or above means this goal is very important to you. The higher your score, up to 12, the more important the goal.

Heart rate and respiratory reserve

If you scored nine or above, the efficiency of your heart and lungs is very important to you. When developing a home fitness program, include exercises that will condition your heart and lungs, such as workouts on an exercise bicycle, treadmill, nordic skier, etc.

Stress and tension relief

If you scored nine or above, you want an exercise program to help relieve tension and probably to help you sleep. Home exercises cannot eliminate the stressful situations in your life, but they can provide a release from general tension and improve your ability to relax.

Energy

A score of nine or above indicates that you are not satisfied with your present energy level. Home exercise will increase your ability to work and play longer than you are able to now and without getting as tired.

Muscle tone and general conditioning

A score of nine or above means you are concerned with sagging, out-of-shape, or weak muscles. Good muscle tone means not only that your body is in good condition but also that you are better able to cope with the stresses of daily life. Improved appearance is another benefit of good muscle tone. If you scored high, refer to the sections of this book dealing with exercise and stretching.

Fat reduction

A score of nine or above means that you are concerned with excess weight and bulges. If you are overweight, don't forget that home exercise alone will not take off enough of the extra pounds. The right course of action is a combination of exercise, which burns calories, and calorie reduction. Certain bulges (hips, thighs) can be trimmed down by exercise. Home exercise cannot change your body type—whether tall and big framed or short and small-boned—but it can make your body look its best no matter what type of build you have. If your score was high, see the sections of this book dealing with diet and nutrition and with stretching and exercise.

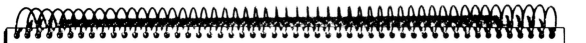

Profile record

Results of Self-Assessments 1, 2 and 3 should now be completed and entered on your "Profile Record." This record can help you assign priorities and determine your most important goals in your home exercise program.

Setting specific and realistic goals is the most important step you can take in developing a successful program because you will have a standard against which you can measure progress. An important long-term goal is to always include exercise in your everyday life. Long after your specific goals have been met, a successful fitness program will help you to remain healthy, trim and relaxed.

Self-assessment 1
What is your attitude toward exercise?

Important attitudes about your exercise habits	Enter your scores from p. 5	Circle if score is 12–10	Circle if score is 9–7	Circle if score is 6–4	Circle if score is 3
		THIS ATTITUDE IS			
IMAGE	_____	Most Important	Important	Somewhat Important	Least Important
ENJOYMENT	_____	Most Important	Important	Somewhat Important	Least Important
APPEARANCE	_____	Most Important	Important	Somewhat Important	Least Important
DISCIPLINE	_____	Most Important	Important	Somewhat Important	Least Important

Self-assessment 2
What is your present level of physical activity?

How active are you?	Enter your scores from p. 7	Circle if score is 12–10	Circle if score is 9–7	Circle if score is 6–4	Circle if score is 3
		YOUR CURRENT LEVEL IS			
EXERCISE	_____	Very High	High	Moderate	Low
ACTIVITY	_____	Very High	High	Moderate	Low
	Total scores of exercise and activity				
COMPOSITE SCORE	_____				

Self-assessment 3
Why do you want to be physically fit?

Important reasons for wanting to be physically fit	Enter your scores from p. 9	Circle if score is 12–10	Circle if score is 9–7	Circle if score is 6–4	Circle if score is 3
		THIS REASON IS			
HEART RATE AND RESPIRATORY RESERVE	_____	Most Important	Important	Somewhat Important	Least Important
STRESS AND TENSION RELIEF	_____	Most Important	Important	Somewhat Important	Least Important
ENERGY	_____	Most Important	Important	Somewhat Important	Least Important
MUSCLE TONE AND GENERAL CONDITIONING	_____	Most Important	Important	Somewhat Important	Least Important
FAT REDUCTION	_____	Most Important	Important	Somewhat Important	Least Important

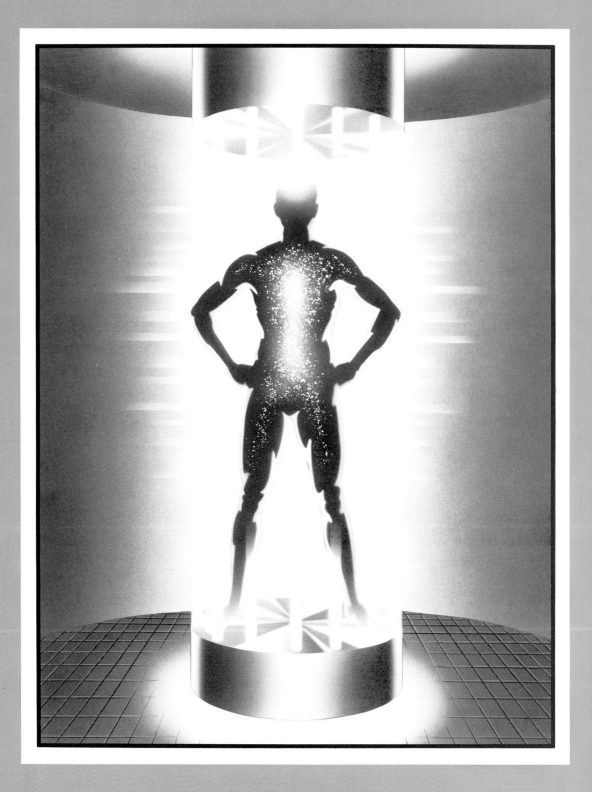

Equipment

The fitness explosion

Over the past several years, the market for home fitness equipment has undergone a renaissance. There has never been a better selection of products or a better time to buy.

On the supply side, a tidal wave of new product introductions by major manufacturers signals a boom market. But competition to move inventory is fierce, and it is doubtful that prices will be this good again for several years to come.

On the demand side, more consumers are buying home fitness equipment than ever before. And there is a new breed of buyer. Whereas, in the past, the main purchasers were younger males, the market has broadened to encompass male and female buyers of all ages. Yes, even pregnant women, the elderly, and your mother have joined the ranks of fitness enthusiasts. National surveys indicate that sixty-five million Americans engage in some form of regular exercise.

Not long ago, if you walked into the average sporting goods store, the selection of home fitness items would have put you to sleep. Cement filled weights, exercise bicycles that looked like they were designed twenty years ago (which some were), weight benches, and a few springy hand grippers were among the typical items that you might find.

Walk into the same store today and you will witness a startling transition. Sleek metalic rowers, shapely inversion boards, space-age antigravity boots, chrome weights, European-designed stationary bikes—and that's just the first aisle!

The reason so many new products are hitting the market is the explosion in demand. Strong sales in the home fitness category are attracting even companies like West Bend and

Campbell Soup. Both are entering the market in a big way. And manufacturers of high-priced commercial gym products, such as Nautilus Sports Medical Industries, among others, are now developing product lines priced for the home.

The upshot is that you, as a consumer, are poised to reap the benefits of these exciting market trends. And *HomeWork-out* will tell you how.

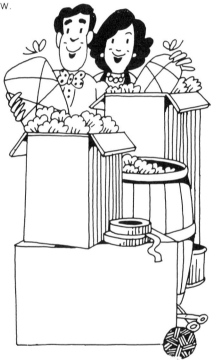

Just looking

If you are not sure what kind of equipment you want, or can afford, start by browsing for ideas, prices, designs, colors, or whatever suits your fancy. If your budget is small, take a close look at the section on "Machines," (see page 34), which contains a selection of inexpensive items that may be purchased through a variety of retail and catalog outlets.

Beyond examining the functional aspects of home fitness machines, try to imagine how

they would look in your home or apartment or where you would set them up. Also, check to see if there are any special requirements for assembly. For example, some devices attach to a wall or floor.

It is usually best to begin buying equipment one piece at a time. By all means, shop around. Check local department and sporting goods stores and even the classified ads in local newspapers for used equipment. You might find a great bargain.

In many cases, manufacturers who sell direct to the consumer offer extended payment terms, and many retailers are willing to set up credit accounts. Another option to investigate is financing your purchase through third-party lenders, such as bank credit cards and independent finance agencies.

Information is vital when you are in the browsing stage. You need as much as possible. In many cases, *HomeWork-out* can direct you to the best possible source: the product maker.

Manufacturers, especially ones who sell directly to consumers, often will send brochures and product information sheets on request. Many have toll-free (1–800) phone numbers. These are included, when available, along with addresses in the listings for each manufacturer.

Quality

The old saying about getting what you pay for was never more appropriate than in regard to home fitness equipment. Another adage to keep in mind is *"Buyer, beware."*

Your home fitness program won't even get off the ground if your equipment breaks down the third time you use it, or if it is too rickety to give you a good workout. The general rule in buying home fitness machines is to buy the best quality that you can afford. This rule translates directly into dollars. If the price on a piece of equipment seems too good to be true, it probably is. Look it over carefully.

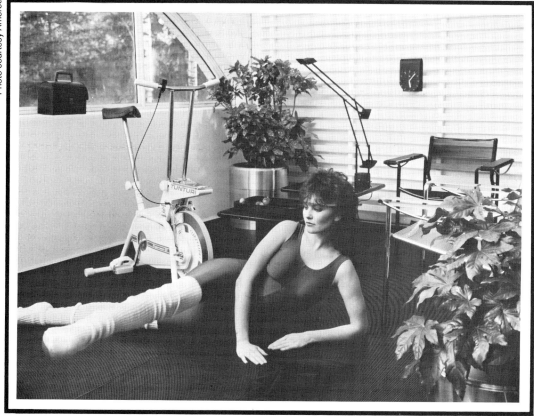

When browsing for equipment, imagine how it would look in your home.

It may not always be easy to spot second-rate workmanship when you are in a retail store, or especially when buying direct or through a catalog. If you are not sure about something, it may help to call (or write) the manufacturer and ask to speak with a consumer service representative.

Here are a few other pointers that may help in assessing the quality of a product.

Materials and construction

Take a close look at the construction of a home fitness machine. If it has tubular steel structure, as many do, how thick is the steel?

Many fitness machines also have a sheet metal framework. How sturdy is it?

If the machine has devices such as a shock absorber-type contraption to provide resistance, test it thoroughly before buying. It is important to determine whether the resistance mechanism will provide enough progressive resistance to allow growth in your exercise program. The same is true of home gyms that use captured weight stacks for resistance. Find out whether the weight stack is expandable.

Also look over any plastic parts, fittings, and coverings for flaws, breakage, or poor workmanship. A quality product generally is made of better materials.

Appearances can be deceiving. A good coat of paint (or chrome) can hide glaring weaknesses in product design and structure. Also, don't be fooled by the machine's appearance into thinking that it *looks sturdy*. If a retail store has a demonstration model, hop on and give it a trial workout. This tactic will tell you more about the sturdiness and function of a machine than a stack of brochures.

Personally testing a fitness machine also gives you a feeling for the compatability of you and the machine. Does it feel comfortable to use? How does it fit in with your personal exercise goals?

In fact, it is a good idea to try out any exercise product before buying. If nothing else, you will know whether the product performs mechanically the way the manufacturer claims. Some don't.

Also look for any tell-tale signs of wear and tear on the in-store demo units. As any retailer will tell you, if a product on display can be broken, a customer will find a way. This test may indicate how durable the machine will be in your own home.

The best product reference, of course, is a friend or neighbor who has used it and is satisfied. Ask around while shopping. And pepper the local sporting goods salesmen with questions about the construction and workings of a home fitness product. You may be surprised by their candid responses to direct questions. They recognize that a well informed, satisfied consumer is their best prospect for a repeat customer.

Where to buy

Once you have made a decision about what you want to buy, the next decision is where to buy it. Your choices are catalogs, local retailers, and ordering direct from the manufacturer. Each choice has its own set of advantages and limitations.

You may be able to save money by shopping around for the best prices on many of the items shown in this book. Most of the price listings in *HomeWork-out* (except products sold direct from the manufacturer)

are based on manufacturers' suggested retail prices, which includes a fifty-percent-plus dealer mark-up. That means dealers add half (or more) of their wholesale price to the price they charge to consumers.

But some fitness machines may be available at lower prices simply because some retailers don't charge a fifty percent mark-up. For example, if you are willing to shop (and can find the merchandise) at a large discount store where retail mark-up is usually much lower, you could reap substantial savings. Of course, you will get fewer services (such as free delivery or assembly) if you base your decision only on price.

In any case, before you buy, carefully examine the product warranty and the outlet's return policy. Find out whether you or the product supplier is responsible for returning defective merchandise for repair or replacement. In some cases, the return policy (or lack of one) could make a difference in where you buy because some suppliers have a better record of customer service than others.

Another factor to consider is the *potential cost* (any possible additional costs over the price charged for the product) of buying merchandise from various outlets. For example, if you buy a product direct from the manufacturer, find out who pays for shipping to your home and who pays for *return shipping* if the product is damaged, flawed, or if you simply are not satisfied. In many cases, it is the consumer who pays shipping charges both ways, but some outlets reimburse certain expenses, such as returns.

Also, find out whether the outlet accepts product returns, in case the item you buy does not meet with your needs. Many outlets allow returns in good condition within certain time limits.

Listed here are a few additional benefits and limitations of buying direct, through catalogs and from local retailers.

■ **Direct from manufacturer:** This choice is easy in many cases because some manufacturers only sell direct to consumers.

Soloflex is one example. However, some manufacturers, such as Nautilus for the Home and The Lean Machine, sell direct and/or through selected retailers and catalogs. If you can't find the product you want locally, your alternative is to order direct or through a catalog.

Some manufacturers who sell direct offer free thirty-day trials and credit payment plans. Some even pay for shipping to and from your home if you decide not to purchase.

■ **Catalogs:** Catalogs also offer home fitness equipment at highly competitive prices. The mark-ups for major retail catalogs usually are under fifty percent. Prices charged by exclusive, specialty catalogs, however, generally are equal to those found in finer department stores.

One potential drawback of catalog shopping is the time and expense of having to return defective goods through the mail or another delivery service. Another is that you can't personally examine the merchandise without ordering it. The product that you get may seem quite different from what you thought you ordered. However, major retail catalogs do stand behind their merchandise, and the largest operations have convenient catalog outlets.

■ **Retail outlets:** Your most likely alternative is buying from a department store, a discounter, or a specialty retailer, such as a sporting goods store. The biggest advantage in taking this route is that quality retailers offer a wide selection of merchandise and good sales support.

Another important advantage is that you can actually try out the product before making a decision. And you still have the option of ordering the product from a catalog or direct, if the terms of sale appear to favor one outlet over another.

But don't assume that all retail outlets are alike in sales and service. Ask about their policy on repairs and returns before buying. Once again, with retail stores, you get what you pay for. Discount stores, for example, are likely to offer the lowest prices and the least service. Consumers are left to their own devices on assembling and caring for the product.

Sporting goods and specialty stores, such as bicycle shops, usually charge premium prices, but product variety, sales support, and service are much better than in discount operations. For example, many sporting and specialty stores offer free delivery and assembly. And some of the most interesting products are available only through these outlets. Many of these stores also will special order products listed in *HomeWork-out,* if they cannot be ordered direct by the consumer.

Quality retailers make it their business to know the merchandise and to satisfy the customer. Most consumers gladly pay slightly higher prices for these services.

The actual retail price of an item may be affected by factors such as the dealer's location, the type of retail outlet, local competition, and generally, by what price the retailer thinks you, as a consumer, will pay. Some retailers can be quite flexible on expensive items, if you like to negotiate.

Buying and using equipment

If you have never before purchased home fitness equipment, it is easy to become confused by the number and variety of products on the market. You may wonder whether you should buy a stationary cycle, a rower, a multi-station gym, or, if you can afford it, all of the above.

While it is nice to have a variety of home exercise machines, it is not essential. You have more to gain by regularly using a single piece of equipment than by giving up on a roomful of the best machines. In other words, fitness equipment does not represent a good *value* for your money unless you use it. Before you buy, make sure that you feel comfortable *using* a machine.

This chapter will give you a few guidelines on purchasing various pieces of home fitness equipment. But the purpose here is not to instruct you on what to buy; it is to show you what general types of machines are available and to help you guide your thinking. As an educated consumer, you will be able to make your own choices.

Following is a list of commonly available products, what they do, and what to look for or avoid when shopping.

Stationary cycles

Stationary cycles are designed to imitate the action of riding a bicycle, but without the bumps, potholes, wind, and natural elements getting in the way. Their purpose is to condition your heart and lungs by making them work harder during regular exercise. As an additional benefit, these machines tone the muscles in your lower body.

All stationary bikes will give you a workout—even the stripped down, cheaper models. But if you buy a cheap one, you might have to put up with a wobbly, noisy contraption that soon loses its appeal. It makes sense to buy the best quality that you can afford, especially if the stationary cycle is to be your only (or main) piece of exercise equipment.

Stationary cycles are available with a wide range of features. However, some costly features, such as ergometers (which provide feedback on your level of exertion), have little to do with the *function* of the exercise bike itself. If your decision on which model to buy is influenced mostly by price, prioritize your selection by looking for features that improve the function of the cycle, such as heavier flywheels and sturdy frame construction. A lower priority, but certainly worth having, are useful accessories such as electronic feedback instruments.

Some stationary cycles also combine rowing and pedaling action to exercise both the upper and lower body. These machines are great, as long as the rowing doesn't interfere with the pedaling. It is possible to duplicate the same exercise on any stationary

cycle by using hand-held weights while pedaling.

Regardless of the type of stationary cycle that interests you, the best way to select one is to test ride models made by several

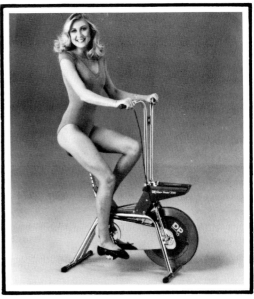

Photo courtesy Diversified Products

manufacturers. If the ride on one model is jerky, or if there are pronounced dead spots in the pedaling action, keep looking until you find one that feels right.

Following is a description of the main components of a stationary cycle, and a few points to consider while shopping.

■ *Flywheels* The purpose of a flywheel is to store energy, which is transmitted through the pedals. The flywheel, in turn, evens out the mechanical action of the pedals. This pedal-to-flywheel action helps to determine the *smoothness* of the cycle's ride, which can make a big difference in the quality of your aerobic workout.

Generally, the weight, shape, and diameter of the flywheel are the main factors that affect its operation. A heavy flywheel made of cast metal (or a weighted wheel) works better than a lighter one (such as a standard bicycle wheel) because it is capable of building more *inertia.* (Inertia is a property of matter that states that an object remains at rest or continues in a uniform motion, unless it is acted on by an outside force.) In less technical terms, it takes more effort to start and stop spinning a heavier wheel than it does for a lighter one.

Likewise, a larger diameter flywheel theoretically provides smoother action than a smaller one of the same weight because its speed around the perimeter is greater at equal levels of force. In practice, however, the shape of the flywheel, its resistance mechanism, its materials and construction, and the overall design of the cycle are *all* factors that affect the smoothness of the ride.

■ *The drive assembly* This includes the pedals, crank, sprockets, and chain (or gear box) drive. Pedals are mechanical,levers that translate the pumping motion of your legs into a circular motion that drives the flywheel.

The pedal crank can be connected directly to the flywheel (usually by a chain), or it can be connected through a series of gears. If the connection is direct, the pedals move continually while the flywheel is in motion. An advantage of direct drive mechanisms is that the continual motion of the pedals helps to even out dead spots (at six and twelve o'clock) in the pedaling action.

If the connection is through gears, or if the crank has a slip clutch, the flywheel continues to turn when you stop the pedals. This is called *freewheeling,* and it eliminates the risk of being struck by, or getting tangled up in, moving pedals. One advantage of gear-driven flywheels is that they are relatively quiet and compact.

Regardless of the type of drive mechanism, as a safety measure watch for how well the drive assembly and the flywheel are enclosed. Clothing or shoelaces could become entangled if working parts are exposed. Be especially careful with open-spoked wheel flywheels, which could be dangerous to children and pets. Wheel covers are standard on many models and are also available as accessories.

■ *Gear ratio* Another point to consider is the gear ratio between the flywheel and the pedals. All things being equal, if the ratio is small (which means the flywheel turns slowly), the ride probably will not be as smooth as cycles with higher gear ratios. In general, the faster the flywheel turns, the smoother the ride. However, the weight of the flywheel should be taken into account when comparing gear ratios. Some heavier flywheels are geared lower than lighter ones.

■ *Resistance* The object of using a stationary cycle is to gradually increase the workload as the condition of your heart and lungs improves. The resistance mechanism is simply a workload regulator. While many resistance devices are available, the type of mechanism you choose is not as important as its ability to provide a wide range of progressive resistance, not just a few tension settings. Tension controls should also be easily accessible.

The basic resistance mechanisms are very simple. They range from caliper units that pinch the flywheel, to roller devices that press against the wheel, to friction straps that run around the outside of the flywheel. Less widespread, but equally effective, are cycles and rowers that are equipped with fan-like blades that use air as their resistance.

■ *Frame* Take special note of the frame's construction. Most frames are made of heavy-duty tubing or rectangular steel, but some are built a little better than others. In general, a frame should feel solid while you exercise, and not shake, rattle, and roll. It should have wide stabilizer bars to prevent side to side rocking, and enough length to eliminate fore-and-aft pitching.

■ *Seat and handlebars* These should be adjustable for comfortable use, and they should not move from side to side or up and down once the screws are tightened. Maximum seat adjustment (seat to pedal in the down cycle) should at least cover the range of the fully extended leg of the tallest and the shortest cycle users. When setting seat height, allow for a slight bend in the knee when the leg is fully extended.

Adjustable handlebars offer flexibility in selecting riding position. Although most people sit upright, studies have shown that increased work efficiency is gained from positioning the body slightly forward (in the racer's position), which helps to overcome dead spots in the pedaling action.

Seat and hand grip comfort are also important considerations if you plan to use your bike often and for extended periods. If a bike's seat and handgrips are not to your liking, you always have the option of replacing them, buying a seat pad, or wearing cycling gloves.

■ *Pedals* Many stationary cycles come with pedals equipped with leather or cloth foot straps. Some cycles have pedals that are comfortable even to bare feet. All pedals do the job, but you may wish to customize your cycle with any of a variety of available pedals and accessories.

■ *Instruments* For most medium-priced cycles, a basic speedometer/odometer, and timer are standard. But for higher-priced models, instrumentation has taken a leap into the computer age. Many manufacturers are now including computerized instruments that give electronic readouts of speed, time, distance, workload, and heart rate. These advanced instruments permit users to track their exercise performance with some precision.

Some cycles include *ergometers,* which are instruments that measure workload. Ergometer readings are easily converted into *calories expended,* which helps in setting exercise goals for more efficient weight management. A simple ergometer is a meter that measures the *power* (in watts) that a cyclist generates while exercising. For example, a 150 pound cyclist generating a continuous fifty watts for one minute burns about five calories.

The technology is proven for most electronic instruments, and reputable manufacturers provide quality equipment. But for the really serious fitness enthusiast who plans to buy a stationary cycle equipped with an ergometer, make sure the unit has been laboratory tested. This is to ensure a small variance between *readings* on the ergometer and *actual* workload.

Rowing machines

A rowing machine may be the only piece of home fitness equipment you will ever need. It simulates the action and benefits of rowing, without the boat and water. By all accounts, rowers are among the most popular fitness products available today. Here's why.

A rower not only provides a good workout for the heart and lungs, its motion stretches and exercises all major muscle groups. And because rowing involves a high-repetition pushing and pulling motion, it is less traumatic to the muscles and joints than many other forms of exercise. Like stationary cycling and treadmill running, rowing also burns a lot of calories, which helps in establishing a program of efficient weight control.

Rowing machines are remarkably easy to use and mechanically simple. Most consist of a seat that moves forward and backward on a rail, and two rowing arms (oars), which are attached to a resistance mechanism. The rowing motion begins with the body in a forward position, arms (and oars) extended, and knees bent to the chest. The user pushes back with the legs (until fully extended) while pulling on the oars. In one fluid motion, the user reverses the action, and returns to the starting position.

Because rowing is an aerobic exercise, you get the most out of machines that are capable of smooth, uninterrupted motion. For this reason, the construction and quality of the seat and oars, and the soundness of the frame, are qualities to watch for when shopping. Following are a few additional points to consider.

■ *Resistance* Most rowers use two hydraulic, shock absorber devices that work something like the ones found on a car. They attach to the rowing arms with movable pins or adjustable knobs. By moving the adjustment knobs up or down the rowing arm, the user is able to vary the mechanical advantage of the oars, thereby increasing or decreasing the resistance.

These shock absorber devices are filled with oil, which acts as the resistance medium. The oil flows from one chamber to another through small valves in response to pressure from a piston rod.

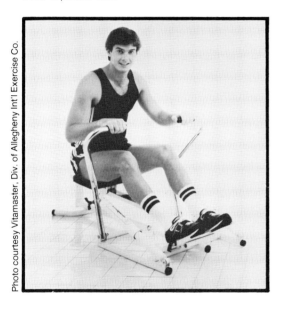

Photo courtesy Vitamaster, Div. of Allegheny Int'l Exercise Co.

One big advantage of the shock-type resistance mechanism is versatility. Many of these rowers are easily converted into compact home gyms capable of a variety of progressive resistance exercises (bench presses, squats, etc.) for both the upper and lower body. Before buying one of these models, however, ask for a demonstration, and give it a try yourself. Try the shock absorbers at several tension settings to ensure that they offer enough range of resistance for growth in your fitness program. Because they are so compact, some of these rower/gyms are a bit awkward to use. But if they feel comfortable to you, they could offer

tremendous exercise versatility and value.

As an alternative to the shock absorber devices, some rowers use a flywheel attached to a pull chain for resistance. One advantage of a flywheel is that it provides more accurate feedback on the level of work being performed, which can be more easily converted into calories expended during exercise. Some purists also claim that the flywheel provides smoother rowing action. A possible disadvantage is that the flywheel limits the machine to one use, *rowing*. But that is, after all, the primary reason for buying one.

■ *Frame* The design and construction of the frame is extremely important. Although most frames are made of steel or aluminum, some manufacturers use heavier-gauge materials than others. The frame should have sufficient length, width (including stabilizer bars), and weight that it does not bounce, creep, or rock during strenuous exercise.

Another factor is frame design. Some frames are built low to the ground for better stability, which may make them difficult for elderly users to get into and out of. Frame length is also a consideration if you are tall. The frame is long enough if all users can fully stretch their legs. Longer frames are also available as options on some rowers.

■ *Oars* These are nothing more than simple levers, but their importance cannot be overstated. Make sure the oars will hold up well under strenuous exercise.

The handgrips can also make a difference. Some rowers have swivel grips, some don't. Some have plastic handles, others have foam.

■ *Seat* The seat, itself, should be comfortable. The best ones have a wide, well-padded, contoured shape. More important, however, is how the seat attaches to the rail, and the type of rail itself, which are factors in the smoothness of a rower's ride. Less expensive rowers have seats that move on twin rails of tubular steel. These seats often have plastic rollers, which are mounted on steel bobbins. About the best that can be said of this construction is that it is functional.

Many better quality rowers have seats that

move on ball-bearing rollers over extruded aluminum rails. On some of these models, the seat rollers are recessed into channels inside the rails, which helps to protect the roller mechanism. Some rowers also have solid monorails, which are sturdy and durable. A nice feature on some rowers is a rubber stop at the ends of the rail, which prevents the jolt of a seat driving into the frame during the stroke.

■ *Footplates* Better quality machines have pivoting footplates, which help to keep the feet in correct position for rowing and other exercises. Footplates should also have adjustable foot straps.

■ *Instruments* To obtain best results from regular workouts with a rower, it is important to measure the approximate work load, the rate of work, and the duration of each workout. In other words, you should know the rower's resistance setting, how many strokes you did per minute (or total strokes), and how long you worked out. Most rowers have markings for resistance settings. Some have built-in stroke counters and timers.

It is also a good idea to keep track of your heart rate while exercising. By tracking the beats per minute, you can estimate your level of work during each exercise session (see *Exercise and Your Heart,* page 160). As you progress in your exercise program, you will be able to increase the work load and the duration of the workout.

Another reason for using your heart rate as an indicator of your exercise level is that it is difficult to accurately measure the work load of rowers equipped with shock absorber resistance devices. Consequently, if a shock-type rower is equipped with an ergometer (a device that measures work load), its readings, at best, provide only work load *estimates.* These readings may be converted into *estimates* of calories burned per minute and total calories expended. Of course, estimates are better than nothing.

Flywheel-type rowers equipped with ergometers, on the other hand, are able to provide more accurate work load readings.

Treadmills

Treadmill running is a pastime that is really hitting its stride. While it is difficult to tell how many of the estimated three million runners in the United States engage regularly in this activity, there is little doubt that the number is growing.

If annual sales of treadmills reflect anything, it is that more runners turn to them as an alternative to being caught in bad weather, nipped by neighbors' dogs, or mugged on the street at night. The benefits of regular workouts on a treadmill are exactly the same as those of running outdoors.

This makes treadmill running one of the single most effective conditioning exercises for the heart and lungs, and one of the best overall methods of weight control. For

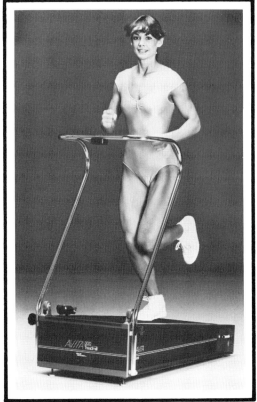

Photo courtesy M & R Industries

example, a 150 pound man or woman jogging on a treadmill at 5.5 miles per hour (an eleven minute mile) burns about eleven calories per minute. At this rate, daily thirty-minute sessions use about 330 calories each, which would allow the individual to lose about twenty-five pounds in a year, or to regularly eat an extra piece of pie or a dish of ice cream with no change in weight.

Treadmills generally are less stressful on the muscles and joints than running outdoors because the running surface cushions and absorbs some of the shock of each footfall. Also, because you remain stationary while running, your body builds no *inertia*. (Inertia means an object tends to remain at rest or in motion unless acted on by another force.) This reduces the stress as your weight is transferred from one foot to another.

Because of these differences between running on treadmills and running the open road, all treadmills will feel slightly awkward to use *at first*. But after a few hours of practice, running on them becomes second nature, so don't be discouraged by your first impressions.

Following are a few additional points to consider when shopping for treadmills.

■ *Motorized treadmills* The biggest difference between motorized and manual treadmills is price. Motorized units may cost several thousand dollars, while the best manual units are generally $1,000 and under. If you can afford the motorized model, it provides several advantages: it maintains a steady pace, which helps in establishing a program of gradual improvement of heart and lung capacity; it automatically moves the tread surface, which makes running a pleasure; and it helps to minimize stress on the feet and legs.

Using a motorized treadmill is easy. After turning the power on and setting the tread speed, you simply step onto the surface and start with a slow trot. With many motorized treadmills, it is not necessary to hold the handrails. After a few minutes of warm-up, you can increase the treadbelt speed on most

models with a fingertip control. When you are nearly finished running, you can slow treadbelt speed for a few minutes of cool-down trotting or walking.

The motors on treadmills usually range between one-half and two horsepower, and they run on two types of electrical current: *alternating current* (AC) or *direct current* (DC). AC motors require less horsepower because they continually run at an ideal speed. Power is transferred to the treadbelt through a belt and pulley system, which usually limits AC motors to a choice of several pre-set speeds.

DC motors are capable of running a treadbelt at variable speeds from zero miles per hour to maximum output. They usually need more horsepower because belt friction places different demands at different speeds. DC motors are preferable to AC, but they are more expensive.

There are also two types of controllers on motorized treadmills: *rheostatic* (also known as potentiometers), and *solid state*. Rheostats, which are found on most AC motors, step down voltage in jumps so the motor can run at several speeds, such as high, medium, and low. They are not very energy-efficient. Solid state electronics, which are found on DC motors, convert standard household current, which is AC, into DC. Along with the controller, all motorized treadmills should have an emergency on/off switch located within easy reach.

A flat running surface is another advantage found on most motorized treadmills. A flat surface is possible because motorized units have enough horsepower to overcome friction. (Most manual treadmills use rollers to minimize belt friction.)

Friction is also a factor in the selection of materials for the treadbelt and the running surface. Motorized treadmills have belts backed with a slippery polyester that moves over flat surfaces made of aluminum, polished wood, or formica. Periodic application of a lubricant (usually silicon) is highly recommended on most models. This helps prevent friction and static build-up.

■ *Manual treadmills* Price is usually the reason for buying a manually operated treadmill. These units are available beginning at prices as low as a few hundred dollars.

Manual treadmills provide the same benefits as motorized models, except that you provide the horsepower by pushing against the running belt with each stride. One consideration when using a manual treadmill is running technique. The motion and force of each footfall should be relatively equal, or the running belt on some models may drift off center, which affects the smoothness of its action. It is also important to concentrate on good posture, as many individuals tend to lean forward.

Most manual treadmills have roller surfaces that minimize belt friction. Regardless of what the rollers are made of (wood, aluminum, etc.) check to see what kind of bearings they have. Smaller rollers, for example, may give the treadmill a flatter surface, but are more likely to have *sleeve bearings* that may require periodic lubrication. (Sleeve bearings look like a tube that fits within a tube.) Larger rollers, which tend to give the surface more of a rippled feel, are more likely to have the preferred ball bearings.

Most manual treadmills also have one or two flywheels, usually the rollers at the ends of the the unit. Flywheel diameter and weight are significant factors in keeping the treadbelt moving at an even speed, especially at the point when both feet are off the running surface.

As final considerations, make sure the running surface is long enough for your stride, and the front and siderails are high enough to grasp comfortably.

One possible drawback of manual units is that they are much noisier than motorized treadmills.

■ *Elevation control* The front ends of most motorized and manual treadmills are adjustable to allow selection of running surface grades from level to steep. The adjustment control should be easy to operate, and lock securely.

■ *Instrumentation* For best results from regular workouts with a treadmill, it is important to measure the running surface grade (elevation), running speed, total distance covered, and the duration of each workout. Most treadmills are equipped with a standard or electronic speedometer/ odometer and timer. Some units include devices that give additional information, such as calories burned during exercise.

Regardless of the type of feedback equipment, it is a good idea to keep track of your heart rate while exercising. You have the option of wearing a heart monitor device, or tracking the beats per minute immediately after you finish. From your heart rate, you can estimate your level of work during each exercise session (see *Exercise and Your Heart,* page 160). As you progress in your exercise program, you will be able to increase the work load (running speed/elevation) and the duration of the workout. Just make sure you don't overdo it.

Trampolines

The trampoline family includes three product categories: full size trampolines, mini-trampolines, and rebound exercisers. Although any of the three could potentially be found in the home, the low cost, safety, versatility and compact design of the *rebound exerciser* makes it the most likely choice for most families and individuals.

Used correctly, rebounders (and trampolines) provide conditioning for the heart and lungs that is comparable to running, rowing, and stationary cycling. Trampolines, however, are unlike rebounders in design and purpose. They are designed to act mainly as springboards for acrobatics, which means that one object of using a trampoline is to get as high up with each bounce as possible. Not only does this require a high ceiling, but it also poses certain risks of injury.

The purpose of a rebounder is to absorb the stress of low bouncing while the user performs a variety of aerobic exercises from a standing or seated position. These exercises help in building strength, endurance, balance, and coordination.

Because rebound exercising is an activity that gets every part of the body involved, it can be the basis of, or an excellent addition to, any home fitness routine. Rebounders may be used with a variety of accessories, such as dumbells, wrist and ankle weights, jump ropes, and more. These accessories add to the aerobic benefits and versatility of a rebounder.

But rebounding does more than just give you a good workout. It's fun. And fun is a

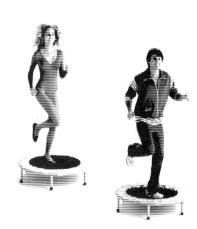

Photo courtesy Diversified Products

commodity that is too often lacking in some home fitness routines. Entertainment can be a factor in motivating an individual to stick with an exercise routine long after his or her initial goals for exercise have been met.

■ *Frame* The sturdiness of the frame is all-important if you plan to use your trampoline or rebounder for years to come. Make sure the materials are durable.

■ *Surface* Rebounders and trampolines come with a variety of jumping mat materials. Make sure the surface is tough, and tear-resistant. Polypropylene, for example, is a heavy-duty nylon material that is favored by several manufacturers.

■ *Springs* Springs on rebounders should be made of tight, heavy-duty steel. They should attach firmly to the ring eyelets (grommets)

that are located around the outside of the jumping mat. As a safety feature, it is also a good idea to buy a rebounder or trampoline with some type of cover that fits snugly over the springs.

■ *Shape* The choices on most models are square, rectangular or round. Square and rectangular units are more stable, and some fold for easy storage. Round models (usually rebounders) are generally less expensive, but they tend to have a soft spot in the center.

■ *Legs* Some rebounders have springy, shock-absorbing legs, which is a nice feature. Others have reinforced, solid legs. The type is not as important as their sturdiness.

■ *Instrumentation* It is a good idea to periodically test your pulse while working out on a trampoline or rebounder. You could buy a pulse monitor that straps to the chest, or, you could simply stop to check your pulse once or twice during exercise. Your heart rate will give you a good measure of your level of workout.

Home gyms

A home gym can make an excellent contribution to any type of fitness program. These gyms are designed to build muscle strength and size, in addition to improving *anaerobic* endurance. (See the section on *Exercising*.)

However, home gyms generally are of only limited help in improving your *aerobic* endurance, which is measured by your ability to do sustained work, such as running or cycling. And aerobic conditioning should be a regular part of your home fitness program. Unless you also run, swim, workout on a stationary cycle (or another piece of equipment that gets your heart and lungs into a sustained level of activity), exercising on a home gym does not give you a complete workout.

One thing a home gym can do, however, is improve your performance in activities that require muscular strength and endurance, for

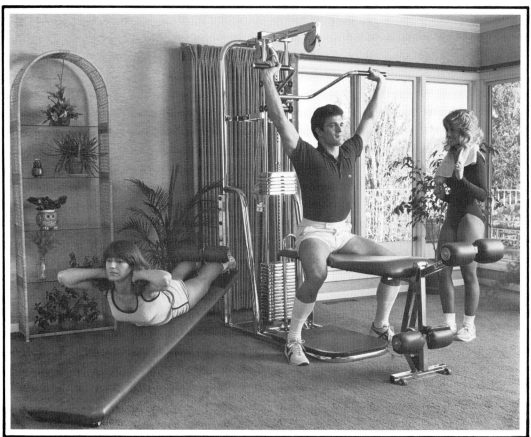

Photo courtesy Universal

instance, lifting a crate into the attic, or carrying a suitcase through the airport. You don't have to be a bodybuilder to derive tremendous benefits from a home gym.

This section lists a variety of home gyms in a wide range of prices and configurations. Following are a few considerations when shopping for one.

■ *Single-station gyms* These are gyms that exercise one muscle, or one specific muscle group. A good example is the Nautilus Abdominal Machine, which performs one exercise extremely well. The biggest advantage of single-station units is that they are uncomplicated and easy to use. Just hop on and exercise, then walk away when you're through.

■ *Multi-station gyms* Most home gyms fall into this category. In effect, these machines are designed to peform a variety of functions, which means that you get more exercise value for your money. A drawback is that multi-station machines may require some preparation, such as switching cables, or moving benches around, when moving from one exercise to another. It is important, if you are thinking about buying a multi-station gym, that you take a close look at the machine's design and functions.

It also is a good idea when looking at multi-station machines to find out what is included in the purchase price. Many units are sold without such amenities as weight benches, and other various accessories that you might think would be included in the purchase price.

■ *Frame* The frame and its support devices are of critical importance to the function of a home gym. In general, the sturdiest frames have the fewest welds. Frames that bolt together have the most potential for shift and wobble.

The quality of a frame's structural materials also is an important factor. But structural materials should be evaluated on the basis of the stresses they will undergo during exercise. For example, a home gym that uses several hundred pounds of cast iron weights for resistance needs a heavier frame than a machine that uses lightweight, elastic bands for the same amount of resistance. When comparing home gyms, make sure you are making real comparisons (apples with apples). And don't forget that a well designed frame made of lightweight materials—aluminum, or smaller gauge steel—may actually be better able to resist structural stresses than a poorly designed frame made of heavier materials.

■ *Resistance* The home gyms found in this book incorporate a variety of different types of resistance: cast iron weights, springs, hydraulic cylinders, elastic resistance bands, and more. And some machines incorporate levers, some use specially designed cams to even out the level of resistance through the exercise motion, and some rely strictly on weights for resistance.

Despite what you may have seen or heard in advertising for these various machines, all of these sources of resistance are capable of producing the desired results of toning and shaping your muscles.

The most important factor is deciding whether the home gym is capable of providing enough resistance for growth in your exercise program.

■ *Materials* As a final consideration, take a close look at the materials that go into a home gym. Are the benches well padded? Is the stitching sound? Does the chrome, or the paint, chip off the weights or the steel tubing? Do you have any options after buying the unit, such as adding on additional weight, or purchasing accessories for new exercises? Let your own good judgment be your guide.

Photos courtesy Soloflex

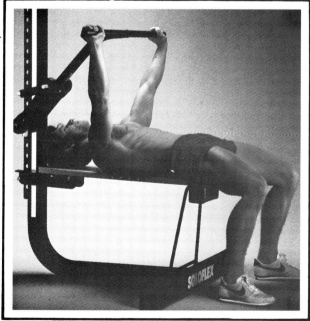
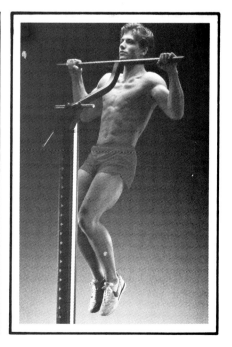

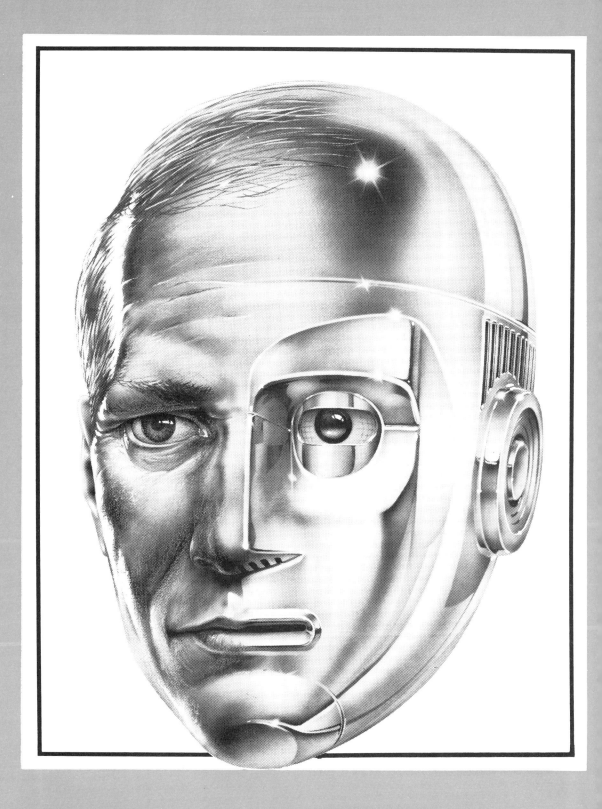

Machines

How to use this section

This section contains selected home fitness product offerings listed alphabetically by manufacturer. A convenient index lists the pages where each manufacturer's goods are located and contains a cross reference of basic product categories, such as home gyms, rowers, treadmills, exercise bicycles, inversion boards, etc.

For example, listings for home fitness equipment made by Diversified Products (DP) are found on page 59. You also can compare each product line made by DP, such as rowing machines, home gyms, and so forth, with the product lines of other manufacturers. Simply consult the ''Product Category Index'' under ''Rowers'' or ''Home gyms'' and you will find page numbers for listings of the products manufactured by AMF American, Vitamaster, and other companies.

Glossary of abbreviations

(')   Feet
(")   Inches
AC   Alternating current
DC   Direct current
COD   Collect on delivery
hp   Horsepower
lbs.   Pounds
LCD   Liquid crystal diode
LED   Light emitting diode
LWH   Length, width, height
mph   Miles per hour

Ajay

1501 E. Wisconsin St.
Delavan, Wisconsin 53115
(414) 728-5521

A major producer of bowling, golf accessories and billiard supplies, Ajay also is building a reputation as an innovative maker of home fitness equipment. All equipment is moderately priced and backed by twelve-month limited warranty.

Exercise cycles

TrimLine Dual Action Cycle   Exercise upper and lower body simultaneously with this flywheel cycle. Handlebars with independent tension control may be moved forward and back while the user pedals. Adjustable pedal tension is applied directly on the axle drum, not on the flywheel. Handlebar height and angle and seat height have quick adjusts. The unit comes with speedometer/odometer and timer, foam hand grips, and pedals with foot straps. Weight: 45 lbs. Color: eggshell epoxy finish. Price: $189.95

Folding Exercycle   This dual action model folds like a scissors for storage. A hydraulic cylinder provides resistance for handlebars, while adjustable tension control on the axle varies pedal tension. Features include adjustable, padded seat, stirrup pedal, and speedometer/odometer. This cycle is constructed of lightweight single tube steel. The folded unit occupies 7½″ × 18″ × 32″ of space. Weight: 18 lbs. Color: eggshell white. Price: $69.95

TrimLine Flywheel Exercycle   This is another dual action bike. Each handlebar has a separate tension controls. The bike has a heavy-duty flywheel with belt resistance system and fingertip tension control. Constructed of sturdy steel tube frame, its other features include quick adjust seat and handlebars, protective chain guard, stirrup pedals, speedometer/odometer, and timer. Weight: 58 lbs. Color: white. Price: $139.95
   The Deluxe Flywheel Exercycle is essentially the same bike with stationary handlebars. Weight: 56 lbs. Price: $129.95
   The 14″ Flywheel Exercycle is similar to the Deluxe Exercycle, with a larger flywheel driven by an elastic drive belt. Tension control is on the pedal axle, not on the wheel. Weight: 51 lbs. Price: $109.95

TrimLine CycleGym   Another model with dual action handlebars, this is the deluxe version of the "Si-

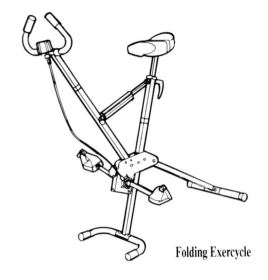

Folding Exercycle

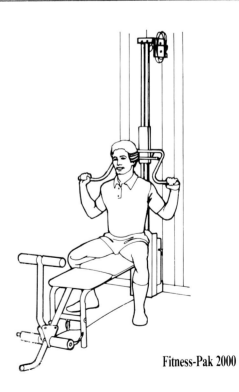

Fitness-Pak 2000

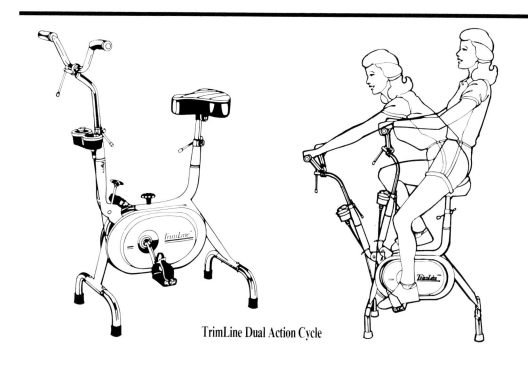

TrimLine Dual Action Cycle

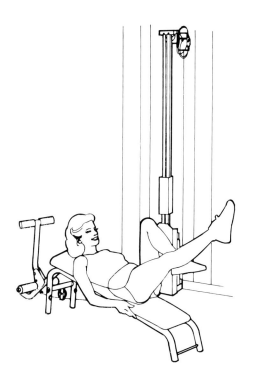

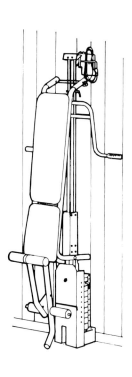

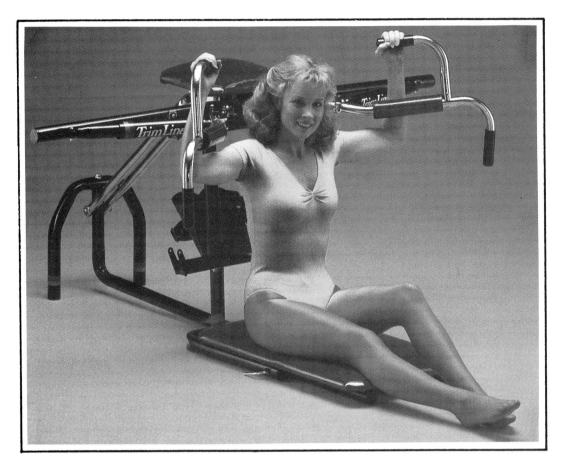

lent Cycle'' line. It has a twenty-inch spoked wheel driven by an elastic belt for exceptionally quiet ride. Tension control is on the axle drum. Features include a steel tube frame, quick adjusting seat and handlebars, speedometer/odometer, and extra wide belt guard. Weight: 37 lbs. Color: caramel with brown trim. Price: $139.95

Three other models in this line are similar to the "CycleGym," but with stationary handlebars. Weight range: 27 to 37 lbs. Color-coordinated finish and tires. Price range: $99.95 to $139.95

TrimLine Exercise Cycles These are three models with caliper brake tension controls and twenty-inch wire spoke wheels. They are chain driven, with sturdy steel oval tube frames, extra large seats, color-coordinated finish and tires, and speedometer/odometers. A timer comes with one model. Weights: 34 and 37 lbs. Price range: $99.95 to $139.95

Home gyms

Fitness-Pak 2000 This is a complete fitness system capable of more than sixty exercises to tone and strengthen every muscle group. Captured weight stack is adjustable from twenty to 110 pounds, with an optional eighty-pound accessory weight pack. A steel weight guard protects hands and fingers. The system includes: press bar that adjusts to high, medium, and low positions; padded exercise bench with leg extension/leg curl assembly; high and low pulley assemblies and cables; a straight bar with hand grips; dual cable hand grips; and a padded ankle strap. The exercise bench is constructed of tube steel with foam padding and vinyl cover, and detaches for use as slant board.

The Fitness-Pak attaches easily to a wall and folds up for flat storage. The unit comes packed in two cartons with weights of eighty and ninety pounds. Colors: black, chrome, brown vinyl. Price: $329.95

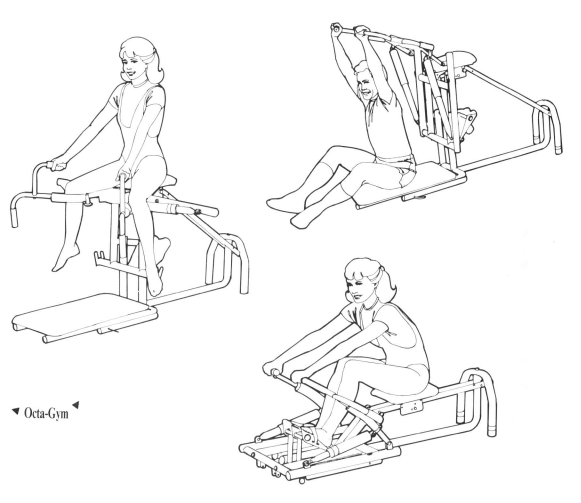

◀ Octa-Gym ◀

Octa-Gym A unique design makes this system versatile and unique. Twin hydraulic cylinders are attached to arms that pivot on horizontal and vertical axles. Adjustable tension settings provide a range of resistance for each arm. In a horizontal position, the system is a rower with a seat that slides on twin chromed steel cylinders. The user's feet are securely strapped to padded rests. Pull up and attach a base unit in vertical position, and the Octa-gym becomes a multistation workhorse capable of press and butterfly exercises for both arms and legs. A red vinyl padded base attaches for seated, kneeling, and standing routines. The user sits on the now stationary rower seat for a variety of leg exercises. The unit is constructed of 1¾'' steel tube with black finish and chromed arms and rails. Weight: 65 lbs. Price: $199.95

Trampolines

TrimLine Jogger Trampoline Three models with different diameters are available. Built of square steel tube with high tension springs and tough polypropylene centers, these trampolines offer durability and lively action. Each has six legs with a choice of screw-on or bolt-on mountings. Protective vinyl covers the springs. Weight range: 21 to 23 lbs. Price: (40'') $59.95; (38'') $54.95; (36'') $49.95

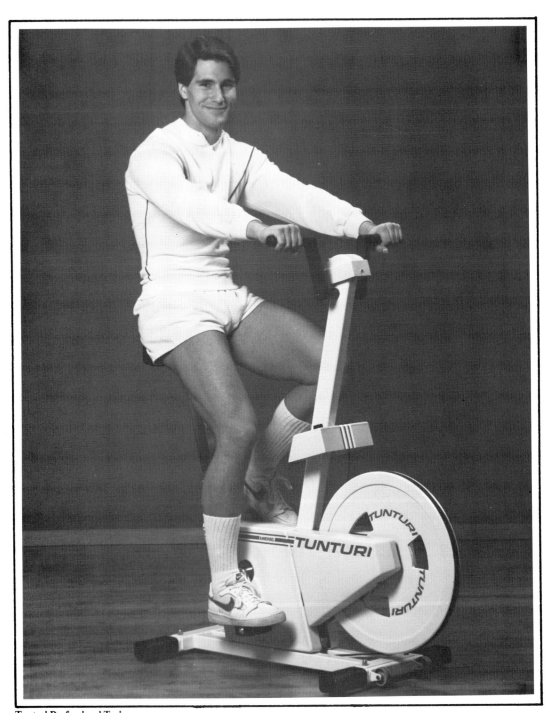

Tunturi Professional Trainer

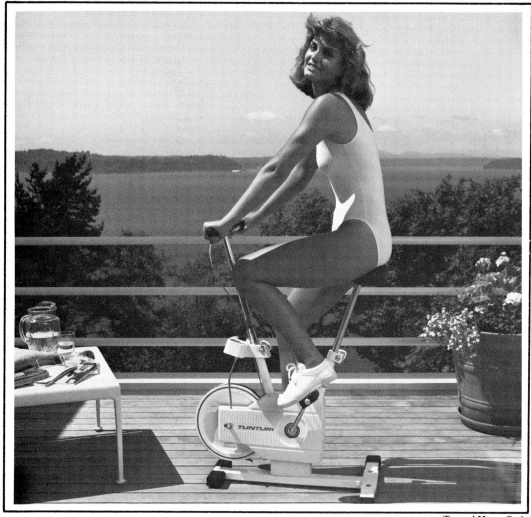

Tunturi Home Cycle

Amerec Corporation

P.O. Box 3825
Bellevue, Washington 98009
1-800-426-0858, (206) 643-1000

Amerec produces quality exercise products in addition to being the exclusive U.S. distributor of Tunturi exercisers, which are among the best in the world. Tunturi products are built in Finland, where harsh winters have led to a reliance on indoor conditioning. Because of favorable (U.S.) currency exchange rates,

Tunturi products currently are artificially low-priced. Call or write for brochures and the location of your nearest dealer.

Exercise cycles

Tunturi Professional Trainer A hefty, fifty-pound flywheel (heaviest on the market) and belt tension system provides ultra smooth operation. Features include: heavy-duty rectangular steel frame; eleven-step workload adjustment; quick-adjusting, foam-grip handlebars; adjustable padded seat; transport

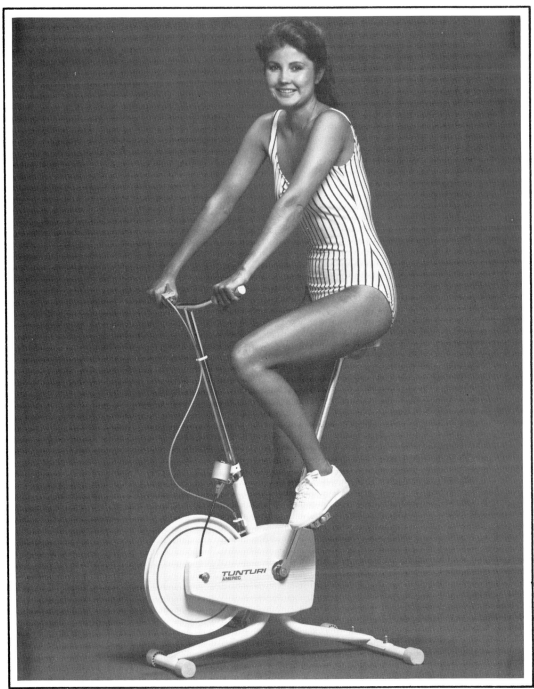

Turnturi Family Cycle

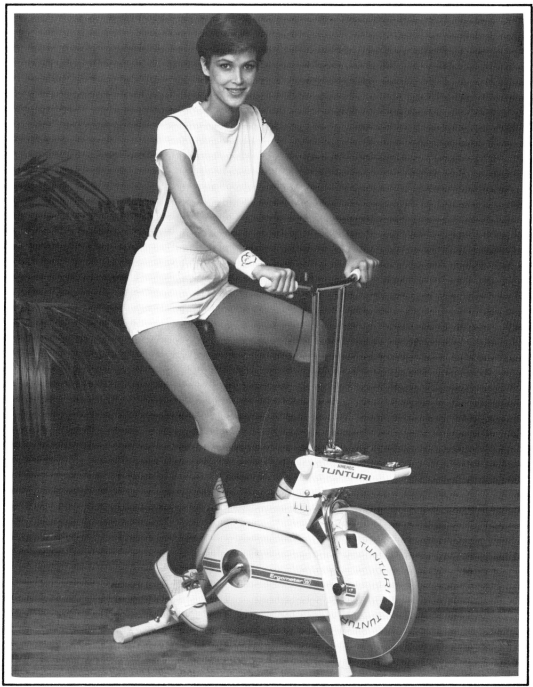

Tunturi Ergometer

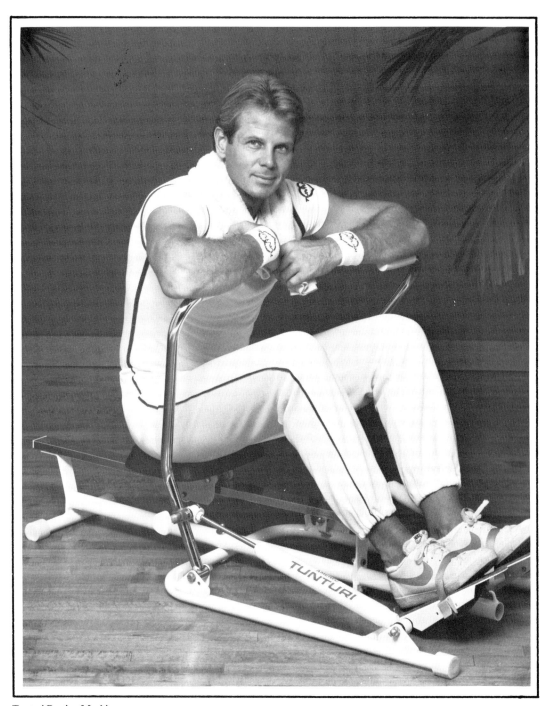

Tunturi Rowing Machine

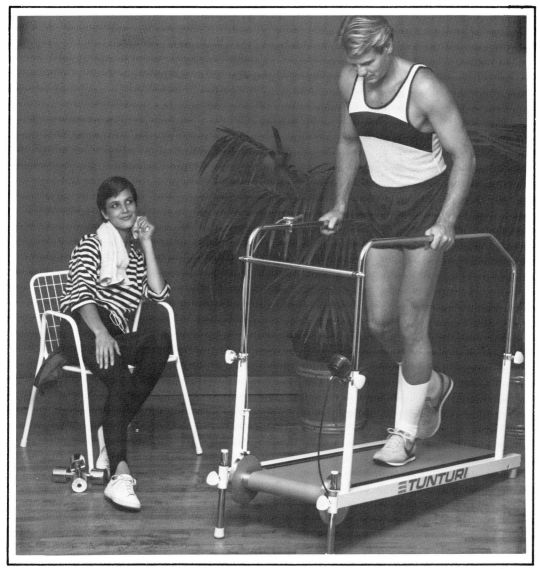

Tunturi Jogger

wheels; and fully enclosed chain drive. The unit comes with tachometer and timer with sound signal. LWH: 43″ × 19½″ × 47″. Weight: 126 lbs. Color: white with green trim. Price: $540.00.

Tunturi Ergometer A heavy-duty tube steel frame with forty-pound flywheel and caliper disc brake resistance system provides a smooth, quiet ride. Features include adjustable, anatomically designed seat; adjustable (forward and back) handlebars with fingertip tension control; pedals with foot straps; and fully-enclosed chain drive. This bike has an instrument panel with tachometer / odometer, ribbon gauge that shows resistance to flywheel (from freewheeling to 450 watts), and timer with sound signal. Optional metronome gives sound and / or light signal (frequen-

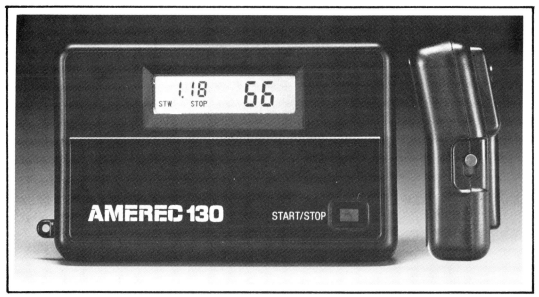

▲ Amerec Pulse Meter, PM-130
This unit features a four-bit microcomputer with built-in quartz clock for a compact, lightweight design that is ideal for jogging, cycling and other active exercise, indoors and out. An LCD digital display indicates pulse rate and stopwatch functions simultaneously. The PM-130 is battery operated with ▶ optional AC adaptor. The unit may be mounted on exercise equipment, or worn on a wrist strap. Price: $119.00.

cies 40–200 per minute). LWH: 37½″ × 20″ × 42½″. Weight: 73 lbs. Color: white with green trim. Price: $349.00

Tunturi Racing Ergometer This is the same basic bike as the Ergometer with racing seat, racing handlebars, and pedals with toe clips. Pedaling resistance is adjustable to twice that of Ergometer (from freewheeling to 900 watts). The Executive Sport model can be equipped with a contest bike's handlebars and seat. Price: $437.00

Tunturi Home Cycle This model is compact and made of sturdy tube and rectangular steel frame. A twenty-seven-pound flywheel has fingertip adjustment of five tension settings. The unit is equipped with an adjustable padded seat and handlebar, speedometer/odometer, and timer with sound signal. LWH: 26½″ × 20″ × 27″. Color: white, green trim. Price: $279.00

Family Cycle This inexpensive bike features a compact design and sturdy construction of tube steel. Features include quick-adjusting seat and handlebar, fingertip adjustment of belt tension system, and speedometer/odometer. LWH: 28½″ × 20″ × 25½″. Color: white, green trim. Price: $135.00

Rowers

Tunturi Rowing Machine 1 An anatomically designed seat moves smoothly on special rollers over a chromed steel rail. Dual, heavy-duty, shock-type cylinders provide even resistance at infinitely adjustable settings. Other features include wide padded foot pedals and cushioned hand grips. LWH: 54″ × 30½″ × 11½″. Weight: 40 lbs. Color: white with green trim. Price: $199.00

Tunturi Rowing Machine 2 A one piece, contoured seat moves on special ball bearing rollers that

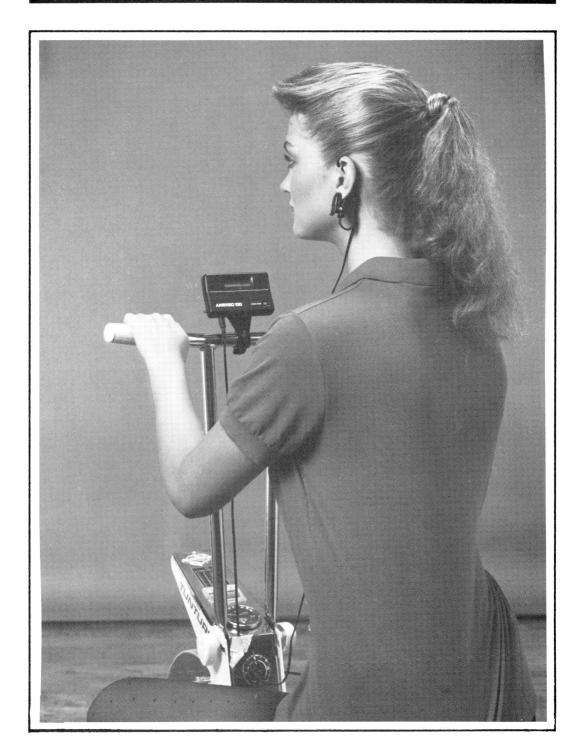

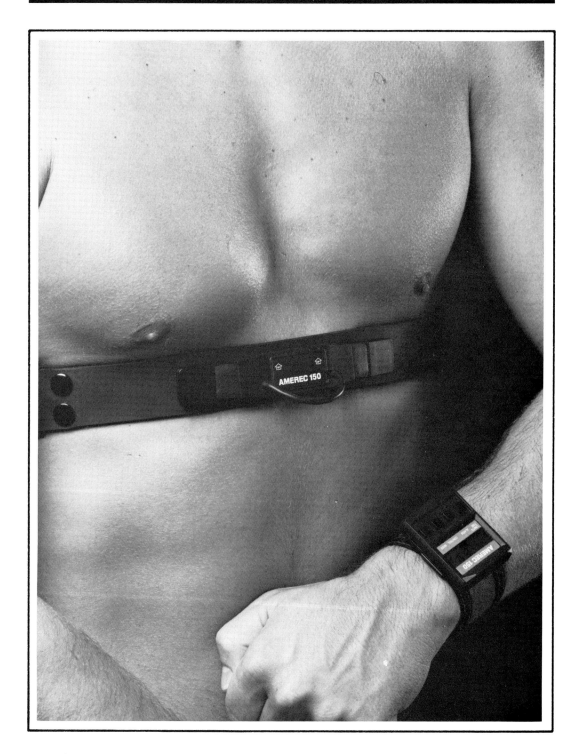

◄ Amerec 150 Sport Tester Telemeter
This monitor transmits heart rate without external wires to an easy-to-read LCD watch panel. The system combines an adjustable chest harness and heart rate transmitter with a compact receiver that can be hand held, attached to the wrist, or to exercise equipment of all types. The 150 can be programmed to help users stay within their training zones by sending an audible signal when the heart rate rises above or dips below preset levels. A memory function allows recall of heart rate over a 64-minute exercise session, in 30-second intervals. The unit also functions as a clock with programmable alarm, and as a stopwatch.
Price: $250.00

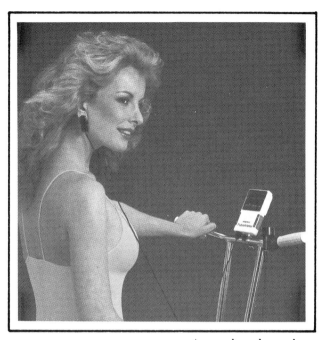

Amerec also makes a pulse meter (model PM-110) with an LED readout. The PM-110 has the same basic functions as the PM-130. Price: $99.00

are completely enclosed in a extruded aluminum rail. Dual, heavy-duty, shock absorber type cylinders attach to rowing arms. Rowing arms feature snap-lock, load adjusters with several tension settings. LWH: 58″ × 30″ × 9″. Weight: 47 lbs. Color: white with green trim. Price: $279.00

Treadmills

Tunturi Jogger This manual jogger has instant workload adjustment control (located on hand rail) that accommodates a variety of body weights and exertion levels. Special rolling bobbins keep the mat centered. The counter-balanced flywheels provide smooth, easy momentum. The running surface adjusts from level to steep incline. The unit comes with height-adjusting side and front handrails and speedometer / odometer. Running range: 42″ long by 13½″ wide. Length: 55″. Mat width: 14″. Weight: 91 lbs. Color: white with green trim. Price: $556.00

AMF American
200 American Ave.
Jefferson, Iowa 50129
1-800-247-3978

Few companies have a better reputation for exercise equipment than AMF American. Its gymnastic equipment was selected for exclusive use in the 1984 Olympic Games in Los Angeles. After more than twenty-five years as a major supplier of exercise equipment to schools, gymnasiums, and colleges, AMF is becoming a force in the home fitness category. Its innovative products and award-winning designs are widely recognized as among the best available.

Exercise cycles

Benchmark 940 Cycle   This breakthrough product is designed from the bottom up. Rather than perching on a hard saddle with pedals underneath, the user exercises from a seated position with the pedals directly in front. A telescoping seat is mounted on an extruded aluminum slide bar that accommodates users up to 6'7'' tall. Resistance is provided by an adjustable electromagnetic system with a heavily-weighted flywheel to add the sensations of mo-

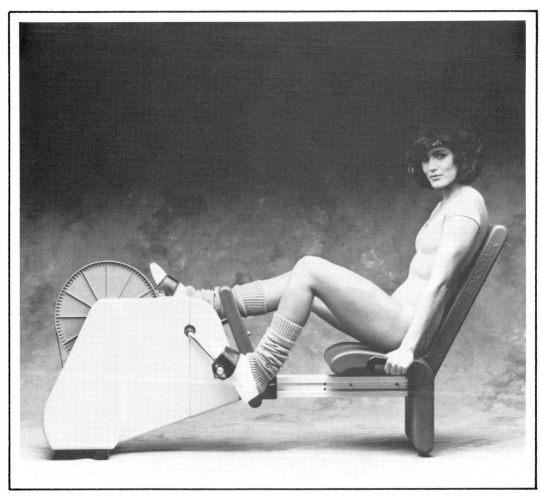

mentum and glide. An on-board computer control panel delivers feedback through an LED readout of time, pedal resistance from one to twenty settings, and calories spent. The electronics are operated by a low-voltage transformer that plugs into a standard wall outlet. Pedals with adjustable foot straps and padded handgrips are placed to provide maximum exercise efficiency. The seat slides in for compact storage, and concealed rollers offer portability. LWH: 62½″–75″ × 17″ × 31″. Price: $695.00

Home gyms

Lifestyler 2000   More than sixty exercises are possible with this versatile gym. The 2000 uses a fulcrum and dual hydraulic cylinders that provide variable resistance with twelve color-coded settings. Because the system is hydraulic, resistance (to maximum levels) equals force exerted by user, from zero pounds almost to infinity. The complete system includes a wall unit with black baked metal finish and bench attachment with reinforced vinyl covering. The bench folds to a width of eighteen inches. A sixty-second timer is mounted in the frame. LWH: 19″ × 34½″ × 73″. Price: $395.00

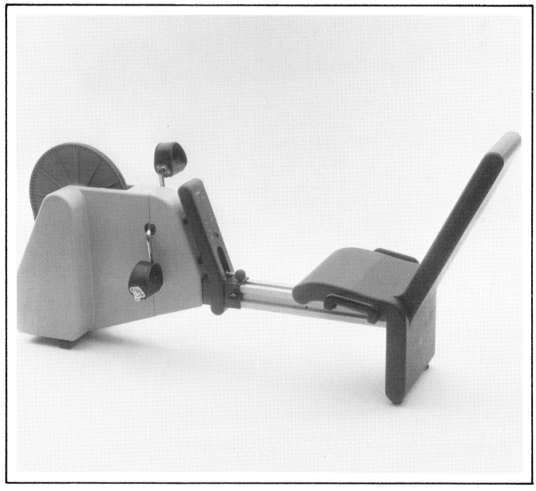

◄ **Benchmark 940 Cycle** ▲

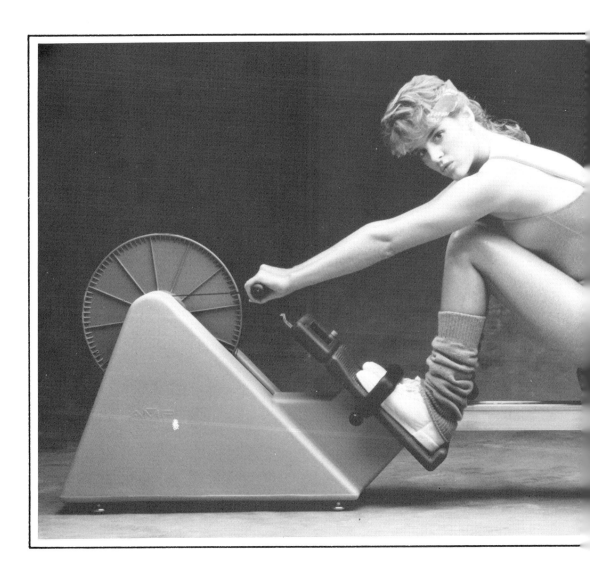

Rowers

Benchmark 920 Rower An award-winning design combined with state-of-the-art electronics makes this rower truly exciting. Using a single, strap-mounted handgrip pulling against a continuously variable electromagnetic system, the rower produces a realistic sculling motion. It lets you develop workout techniques such as biceps curls, reverse curls, and rowing to one side at a time. Resistance is adjustable up to one-half horsepower in twenty increments. On-board computer control delivers feedback through an LED readout of time, resistance, and calories spent. The electronics are operated by a low-voltage transformer that plugs into a standard wall outlet. A telescoping, padded seat is mounted on an extruded aluminum slide bar that accommodates users up to 6'7" tall. The unit comes with adjustable, contoured foot-retainers. The drive mechanism and flywheel are protected by high-impact molded housing. LWH: 82½" X 14" X 25½". Weight: 74 lbs. Price: $595.00

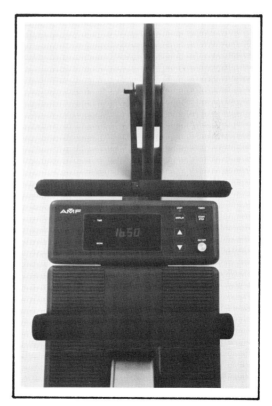

◄ **Benchmark 920 Rower** —**AMF American** ▲

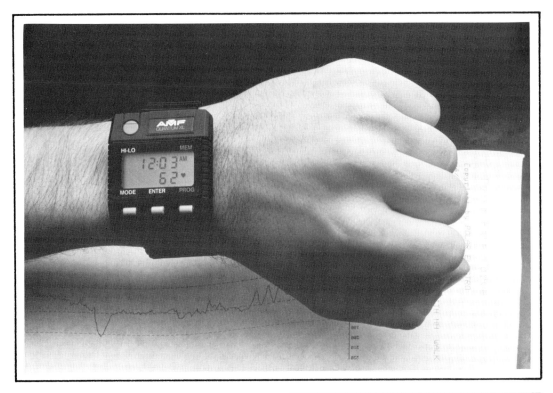

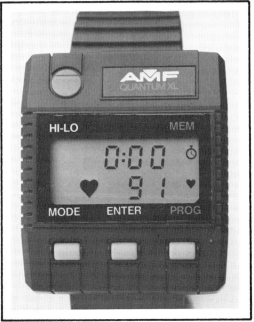

Benchmark Quantum XL Fitness Monitor
One of the most advanced sports/fitness monitors, the XL is designed as a technological aid to exercise. Adjustable chest strap has carbon electrodes that monitor the heart's activity. Information is transmitted to a wristwatch, where heart rate is displayed. A program button allows monitoring of time, time and pulse, stopwatch and pulse, and pulse memory recall. High and low alarms help keep the user in target heart rate zone. Pulse memory keeps track of heart rate at programmable stages of exercise (for example, every five seconds for one hour and twenty minutes). This is an invaluable aid during for post-exercise analysis, and for those who want to know more about their bodies and body functions. Price: $295.00

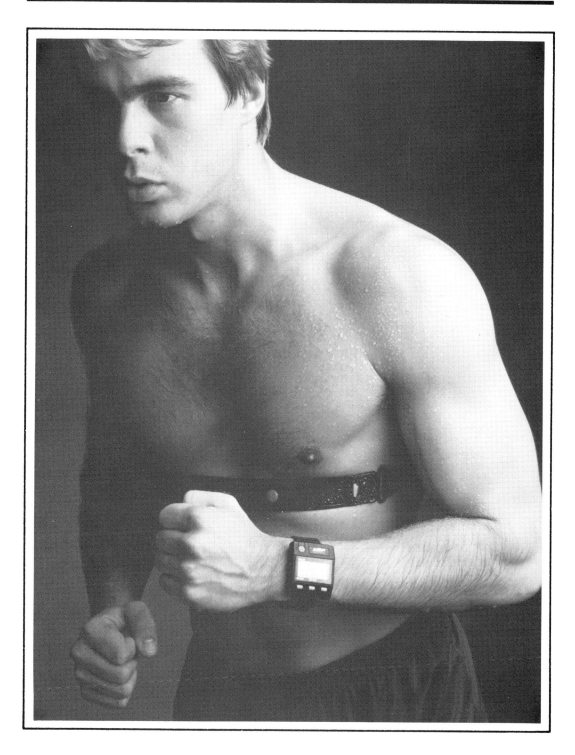

Concept II, Inc.

RR 1, P.O. Box 1100
Morrisville, Vermont 05661-9727
(802) 888-4404

Concept II is a small manufacturer that makes one of the most unique rowing machines available. With a growing following of amateur and professional athletes, health clubs, exercise trainers, and now, home fitness enthusiasts, this low-key company has found an unusual niche in the market. Evidence of loyalty to its product-the Concept II Rowing Ergometer-is easy to find. Various clubs have organanized indoor rowing regattas using the Concept II. These competitions each year attract hundreds of participants from all walks of life. For example, a recent regatta in Boston attracted over 500 participants. For more information about the company and its products, write or phone for free brochures and the company's newsletter.

Rowers

Concept II Rowing Ergometer   Used by competing oarsmen for off-water training, this rower closely simulates the smooth action of rowing. To begin the stroke, the user pushes with the legs, sliding back on a contoured seat that is mounted on a stainless steel monorail with ball bearing rollers. The back and legs work together through the middle of the stroke, and the upper body completes the stroke with a hand-held pull chain. The pull chain returns automatically to start position and draws the user forward, ready for the next stroke.

A flywheel equipped with plastic fan blades provides air resistance. The action of the flywheel simulates the momentum of a boat moving through water. Air resistance increases or decreases-like the drag of water-as a function of the speed of rowing. Resistance also may be altered by moving the drive chain to engage various sized sprockets, which change the user's leverage on the flywheel. These resistance options enable the user to develop workouts for both aerobic and anaerobic conditioning.

Measuring exercise performa ce is accurate and easy with an attached speedometer/odometer, and a wrist watch. Exercise data is easily converted into calories burned per hour. An optional computer program (for the Commodore 64) is available to perform calculations for the user. The program also creates racing simulations, which provide incentive for using the machine. Program and parts are $60.00.

The unit has an overall length of 100″. By removing four bolts, it is collapsible to a length of 60″. Height: 34″. Width: 18″. Shipping weight: 78 lbs. Partial assembly required. Price: $595.00. Shipping cost range: $10.00 to $39.00, paid C.O.D. Orders may be paid by check, money order, or C.O.D.

A note on prices

Prices listed in *HomeWork-out*—with the exception of products sold direct from the factory—are manufacturers' *suggested retail prices,* and may not reflect the true cost of purchasing home fitness equipment in your area. By federal law, retailers are free to set their own prices. So don't be surprised if the cost of an item to you is higher or lower than the suggested retail price.

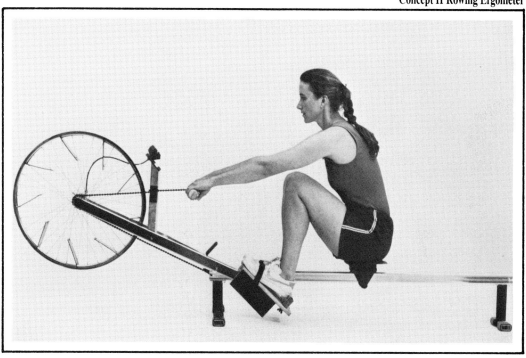

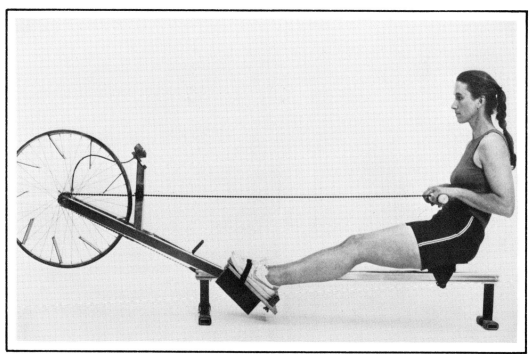

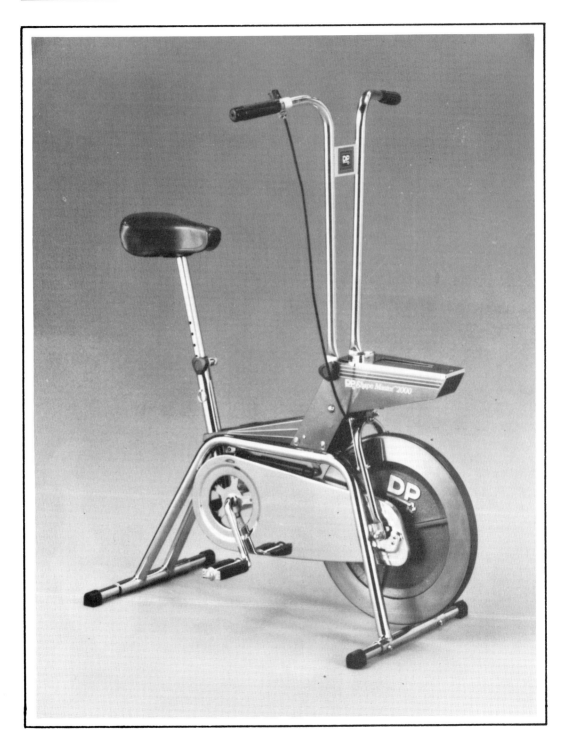

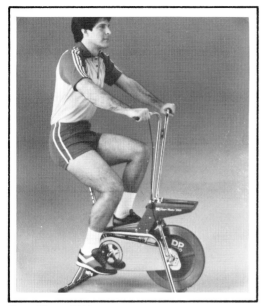

◄ Shape Master 2000 ▲

Diversified Products (DP)
P.O. Box 100
Opelika, Alabama 36802
(205) 749-9001

By far the largest manufacturer of home fitness equipment, DP also is a leading advocate of physical fitness for everyone. With its "Fit for Life" advertising campaign, the company is spending multiple millions each year to say that fitness builds strength, energy, and an attractive appearance. You've probably seen and heard DP's ads. It's a good idea to look at DP's equipment.

Exercise cycles

Shape Master 2000   A lot of bike for the price, the 2000 features a thirty-nine-pound flywheel for free-wheeling effect; a heavy-duty chromed, tube steel frame; and a caliper disc brake system with fingertip tension adjustment. Other features include a low center of gravity for stability, adjustable handlebars and seat, enclosed chrome chainguard, and padded seat. The instrument console contains tension gauge, speedometer, odometer, and timer. Colors: red, grey, black. Price: $299.00

Body Shaper   This bike features a fifteen-pound flywheel, a chromed tube steel frame, and caliper brakes with infinite tension adjustment. Other features in-

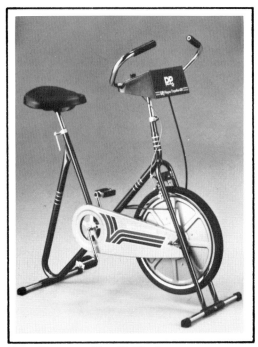

Fitness Express —Diversified Products

clude twin adjustable handlebars; enclosed chain; twenty-inch bicycle wheel with molded covers; ball bearing pedals; and padded, adjustable seat. The contoured instrument console contains speedometer, odometer, and timer. Color: chrome, charcoal grey and red. Price: $159.00

Fitness Express   This bike has a steel tube frame; caliper brakes with infinite tension adjustment; enclosed chain; adjustable seat and handlebars; twenty-inch bicycle wheel with molded cover; and an instrument console with speedometer, odometer, and timer. Color: charcoal grey and red. Price: $149.00

DP Mark 1   This instrument is similar to the Fitness Express, with a different speedometer, odometer, and timer, among other minor variations. Price: $139.00

DP Pacers (300 Deluxe, 250, 200)   These are budget models, but all have the same heavy-duty steel frames found on more expensive DP bikes. The 300 Deluxe and the 250 have twenty-inch bicycle wheels and caliper tension controls. The 200 has a twenty-inch bicycle wheel and a roller-type tension control. All three models have ball bearing pedals, adjustable seats and handlebars, enclosed chains, speedometer, odometer, and timer (no timer on the 200). Price range: $89.00 to $99.00

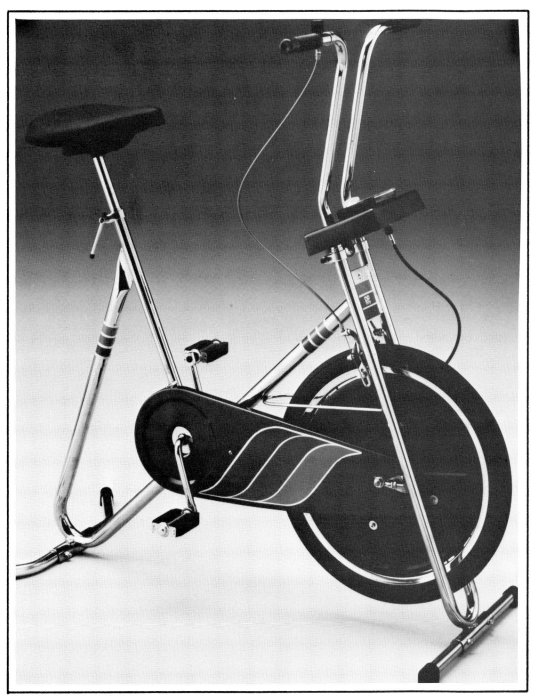

Body Shaper —Diversified Products

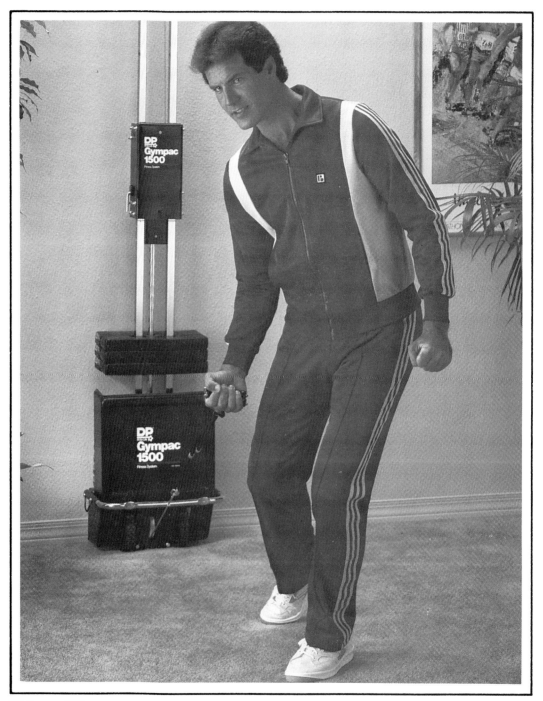

DP Gympac 1500

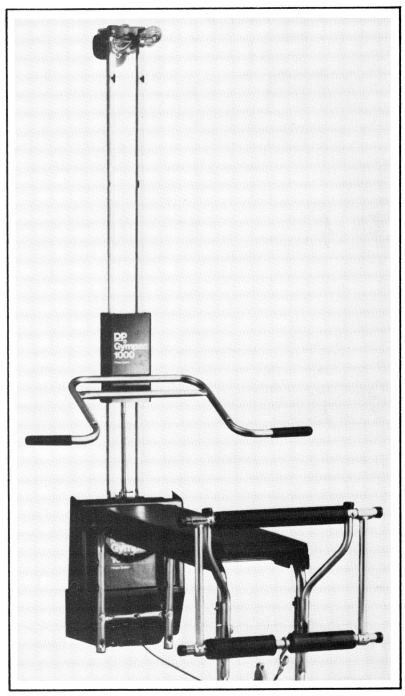

DP Gympac 1000

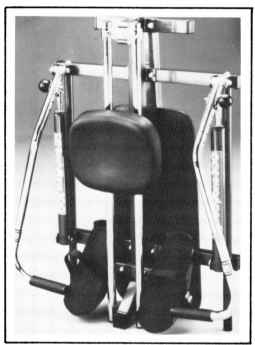

BodyTone 300

DP Gympac 1500 This is the deluxe model of DP's home gym line. With accessories, the Gympac 1500 is capable of all major barbell and pulley exercises. Gympac comes with 110-pound weight stack with optional eighty-eight-pound accessory pack. For safety, weights slide on twin steel beams; a weight guard prevents pinched fingers. A handlebar with revolving hand grips adjusts to six positions for a variety of exercises from bench presses to chin-ups.

The weight bench includes a padded leg lift/leg curl/rowing attachment. The padded bench inclines for sit-ups (foot strap included). Leg cuff, pull bar, and twin hand grip attach to pulleys at the top and bottom of the Gympac unit for arm and leg exercises.

Wall-mounted, the Gympac may be released from mountings by removing a single wing nut. It rolls to storage on permanent rubber wheels. An optional stand makes Gympac free-standing.

LWH (including bench): 53″ × 38″ × 85″. LWH (folded for storage against wall): 17½″ × 38″ × 85″. Color: black, chrome, metallic-flecked red vinyl. Price: $299.00

DP Gympac 1000 This gym has the same design and most features of the Gympac 1500. An important difference is that Gympac 1000 comes with a double leg extension device that does not have a leg curl/rowing feature. However, a deluxe leg lift/leg curl/rowing attachment may be purchased as an accessory. A minor difference is black vinyl covering instead of red. Price: $269.00

DP Gympac Systems This family of modular, wall-mounted exercise units is similar to equipment found in health spas. The family includes a Bench Press Module, a Leg Lift/Leg Curl Module, and a Wall Pulley Exerciser. Each machine focuses on specific muscle groups and each comes with weights that glide up and down on twin steel beams. Accessory weight packs containing five 11-pound weights may be purchased for any unit. All machines fold up for compact storage.

The Bench Press has a forty-seven-inch locked-in-place foam-padded bench that converts to a slant board. It comes with ten 11-pound weights and chrome handlebars with revolving grips and crossbar. Price: $199.00

The Leg Lift/Leg Curl machine comes with a thickly padded apparatus that attaches to the pulley system and five 11-pound weights. The padded table is bolted to wall unit for sturdy support. Price: $199.00

The Wall Pulley, which is especially suited to women's exercises, includes top and bottom pulleys, long and short bar with hand grips, ankle cuff, double handle rope assembly, and five 11-pound weights. Price: $199.00

Rowers

BodyTone 300   This machine converts from a conventional rower in the horizontal position to a multi-gym when turned vertically. Capable of a wide range of exercises for the upper and lower body, the BodyTone 300 has twin arms and dual hydraulic cylinders with six tension settings. A versatile padded bench attaches in different positions to allow pullovers, bench press, and other exercises. A tele-scoping frame permits adjustments for leg length when used as a rower. Other features include handles with revolving grips, molded contoured seat, and padded footrests with straps. The unit is constructed of 1¼'' round and 1½'' square steel tube. Assembly required. Weight: 49 lbs. Maximum usage position: 49'' long, 30'' wide, height will vary with user. LWH (for storage): 34½'' × 30'' × 9''. Color: chrome, metal grey. Price: $179.00

Trampolines

DP Indoor Jogger   This trampoline features six-leg, all-steel frame; thirty-two steel springs; thirty-six-inch diameter, heavy-duty nylon rebound surface; and vinyl-covered polyfoam padding around edges. Price: $29.99

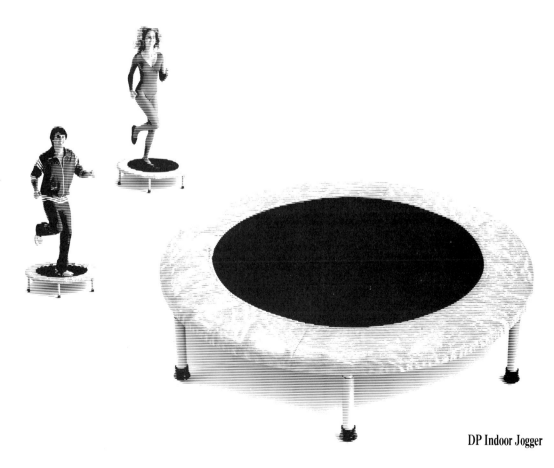

DP Indoor Jogger

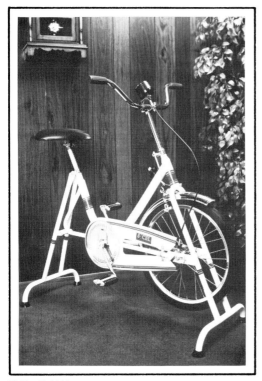

Helios E-2000

Excel

Division of Rocket Industries
9935 Beverly Blvd.
Pico Rivera, California 90660
1-800-392-2258, (213) 699-0311

A leading manufacturer of home fitness equipment, Excel offers good quality at reasonable prices. The company also produces a complete line of weight benches and hand-held products. Call for free brochures. Send $1.00 for a catalog and the name and address of the nearest dealer.

Exercise cycles

Helios E-2000, E-2002   These are basic bikes. The E-2000 has quick adjusts for seat and handlebars, a twenty-inch spoke wheel, fully enclosed chain, and a caliper resistance system with knob control. The unit comes with speedometer/odometer. A 1¾" tube steel frame comes with white finish and chrome fender.

The E-2002 has the same frame and features with a few extras, including covered wheel with solid rubber tire, deluxe padded seat and handlebars, and sixty-

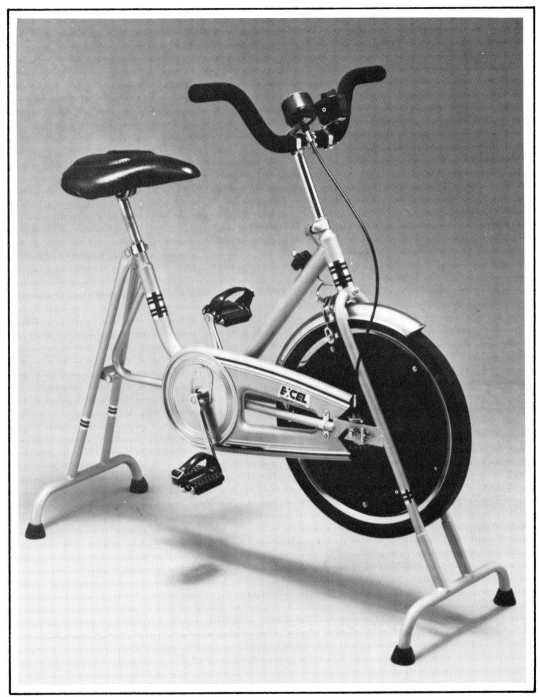

E-2002

minute timer. It is finished in silver with black and chrome foil. Price: (E–2000) $99.95; (E–2002) $119.95

E–3000 Flywheel Exercise Cycle A fifteen-pound flywheel and adjustable belt tension control gives smooth, trouble-free performance. The bike has quick adjusting padded handlebars and seat, non-skid foot pedals, and fully enclosed chain drive. Instruments include speedometer/odometer and timer in a compact console. The E–300 is constructed of heavy-duty tube steel with black finish and silver accents. Price: $139.95

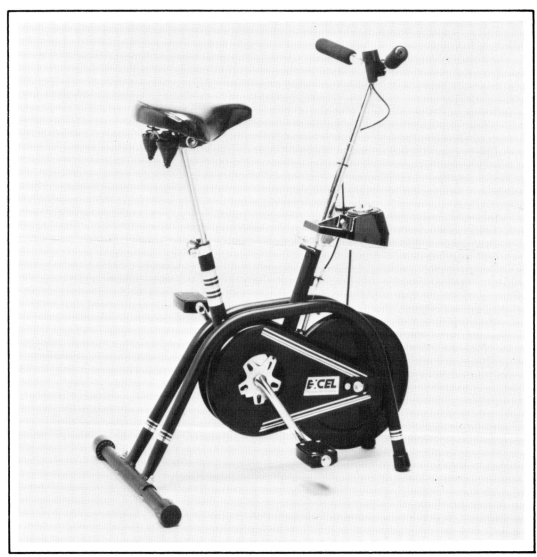

E-3000 Flywheel Exercise Bicycle —Excel

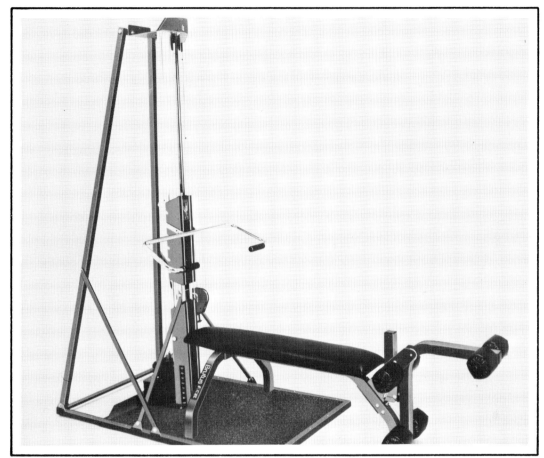

Body Tech Home Gym

Home gyms

BodyTech Home Gym 1000   A versatile home gym that can be wall-mounted or free-standing with an optional frame, the 1000 is capable of thirty-six exercises for development of all muscle groups. With the purchase of optional sidebar, padded leg developer, and padded exercise bench, the system becomes a complete fitness center. The basic system has a carpeted base for standing or seated exercises, a ten-position lifting bar, and a 100-pound captured weight stack in ten-pound increments (expands up to 340 pounds). Additional weights are available in ten-, twenty-, and thirty-pound increments. The system also features ball-bearing pulleys, polyurethane rollers, shock-absorbing weight bumper pads, weight shield, sponge rubber hand grips, double hand cables, and padded ankle strap. The finish is available in rust or black and chrome. Price: (base unit) $699.95; (with frame) $799.95; (frame only) $149.95; (accessory weight set) $59.95

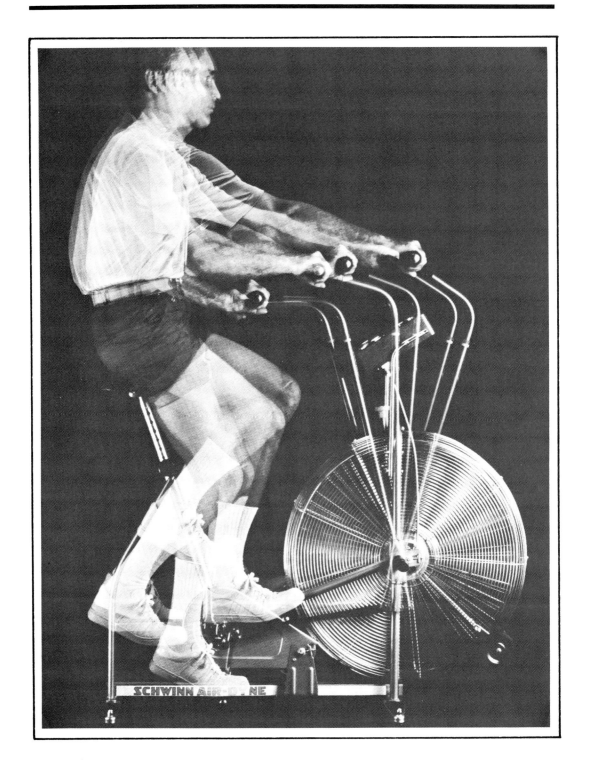

Excelsior Fitness Equipment Co.

Division of Schwinn Bicycle Co.
615 Landwehr Road
Northbrook, Illinois 60062
1-800-228-2222; 1-800-642-8788 (in Nebraska); (312) 291-9100

Excelsior sells only through authorized Schwinn dealers. Its products are guaranteed to be free of defects in materials and workmanship by Schwinn's "no-time-limit" warranty. Call for free brochures or for the name of the dealer nearest you.

Exercise cycles

Schwinn Air-Dyne The Air-Dyne is one of the most distinctive bikes on the market. Utilizing an exclusive air displacement wheel (essentially a fan) for resistance, the bike exercises upper and lower body separately or simultaneously. Pedaling and/or pushing and pulling on arm levers starts the wheel moving, which creates drag (wind resistance). As the user works harder, the wheel turns faster, generating more resistance and a breeze that cools the operator. A console includes a digital countdown timer with audible alarm, a workload indicator, cumulative odometer, and resettable "trip" odometer.

The Air-Dyne is made of heavy-duty steel tube with adjustable, padded seat; fully enclosed chain and air displacement wheel; padded handgrips; padded foot rests; transport wheels; and heavy-duty pedals. Colors: harvest gold or white. Accessories include a wind deflector and a reading stand that mounts between arm levers. Price: $595.00

Schwinn XR-8 The XR-8 is a more traditional bike that uses a heavy flywheel and caliper resistance system. A convenient knob on the instrument console controls workload levels. The console includes timer with alarm, speedometer, and odometer. The XR-8 features box beam frame construction, fully enclosed chain, pedals with straps, adjustable seat and handlebars, and cushioned seat. Colors: harvest gold or white. Price: $249.95

Schwinn Bio-Dyne Ergometer Engineered for laboratory accuracy, Bio-Dyne features caliper brake resistance with a hydraulic workload measurement system. The system enables the user to select from three pedal speeds—sixty, seventy, and ninety rpms—and adjust the resistance dial to provide equal workloads at each speed. An optional laboratory quality calibration kit with full instructions ensures accurate instrument readouts. Bio-Dyne's instrument cluster shows time, speed (over the road and pedal), trip-meter, odometer, and workload indicator. The bike features adjustable, padded seat and handlebars, box beam frame, smooth pedaling action, heavy-duty pedals with straps, and a steel chain guard. Color: white. Price: $495.00; (calibration kit) $39.95

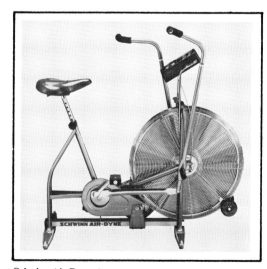

◄ Schwinn Air-Dyne ▲

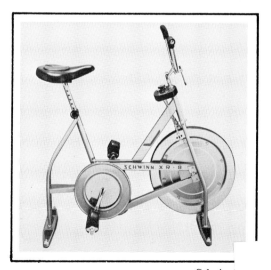

Schwinn

Machine:

Fitness Master, Inc.

1387 Park Road
Chanhassen, Minnesota 55317
1-800-328-8995, (612) 474-0992

This company makes cross-country skiing simulators that are rated by enthusiastic users as the ultimate machines for aerobic conditioning. The company sells direct to customers and accepts major credit cards and COD orders. A no risk, thirty-day home trial is available. If you are not satisfied, the company returns your money and even pays for shipping both ways. There is a two-year warranty on parts and labor. Call or write for brochures.

Cross-country skiers

LT-35 This unit is easy to use: just step on two cushioned foot pads and move your legs back and forth in a scissors motion while pushing and pulling on ski pole-like arms. The machine provides adjustable resistance for both forward and backward motions of poles and foot pads. LT–35 has a chrome-plated steel frame that rests flat on the floor, polymer pulleys and rollers, and heavy-duty cables. The unit is shipped fully assembled. Operating length is 52″. Arms fold down, making unit 5″ high by 24″ wide for storage under a bed. Weight: 31 lbs. Price: $379.00 plus $14.00 shipping.

XC-1 This machine is a deluxe skiing simulator with a design and features similar to those of the LT–35. It is made of the same quality materials with an added feature of two siderails with adjustable pole handles mounted on roller carriage assemblies. The pole handles, which have independent tension adjustments, slide forward and back on rollers to simulate poling. The sturdy siderails are sloped and adjustable to any height. Handles fold down for easy storage five inches high by twenty inches wide. Shipped fully assembled. Operating length is 58″. Weight: 68 lbs. Price: $529.00 plus $20.00 shipping.

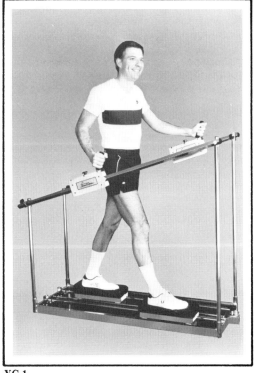

XC-1

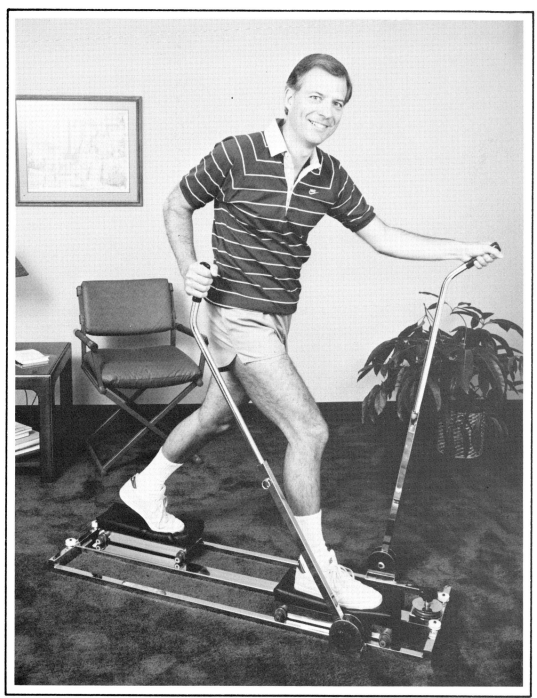

LT-35

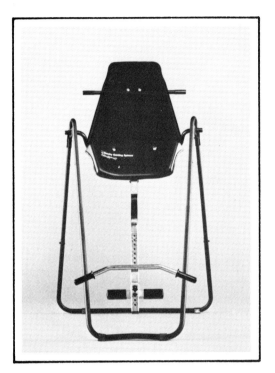

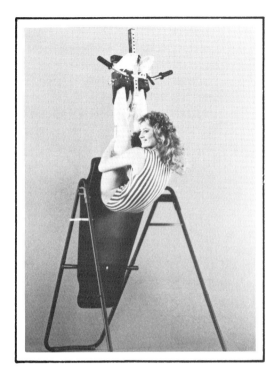

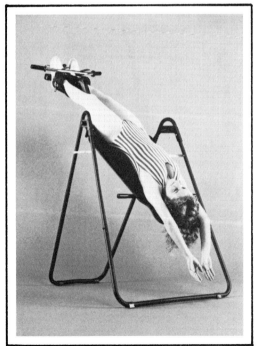

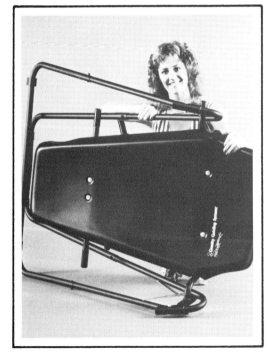

Gravity Guidance, Inc.

1540 Flower Ave.
Duarte, California 91010
1-800-558-1792, (818) 303-4777

The Gravity Guiding System,® invented by Robert M. Martin, M.D., is designed to reverse the negative effects of gravity's constant downward pressure on the body. Gravity Guidance, Inc., offers a series of products based on Dr. Martin's designs, that generate a decompressive force on the muscles and joints by altering body positions through inversion exercise. These products also are designed to improve strength and flexibility with regular use. Best of all, they are easy to get the hang of using. All products feature a patented gooseneck assembly that acts as an automatic compensator for user height and weight. For more information, contact the manufacturer.

Inversion devices

Gravity Guider Series® These inversion devices offer something for everyone. Although each provides for intermittent traction through oscillation, and continual traction through full inversion, the products feature a range of options and prices that make them affordable and versatile.

1103 Series A wide-standing, black, powder-coated "A" frame made of 1" tube steel makes the 1103 sturdy and functional. A comfortable, contoured plastic bed wipes clean after use. Height and weight adjustments for individuals 5' to 6'6" and from 100 to 500 lbs. Rubber coated stop bars and sealed, self-lubricating nylon bearings keep operation smooth, quiet, and maintenance free. Folds for compact storage. $399.95

◄ **Gravity Guider Series 1103**

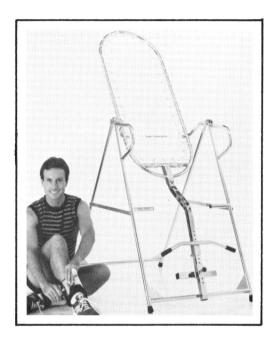

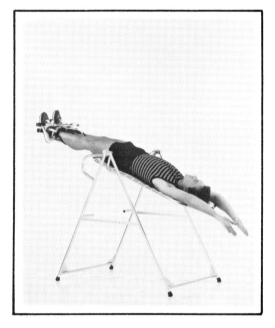

1120 Series This unit is very popular with athletes and regular inversion exercise users because of its sturdy, comfortable design. Made of a 1″ chrome-plated steel tube "A" frame, the 1120 has a wide footprint for maximum stability, and a bed made of tough, vinyl-coated canvas. The 1120 is designed for complete inversion exercise programs, including weight training. A nice feature is the built-in hand grips for mounting and dismounting. (Same height/weight adjustments as 1103 Series.) Folds for storage. Price: $899.95

A note on prices

Prices listed in *HomeWork-out*—with the exception of products sold direct from the factory—are manufacturers' *suggested retail prices*, and may not reflect the true cost of purchasing home fitness equipment in your area. By federal law, retailers are free to set their own prices. So don't be surprised if the cost of an item to you is higher or lower than the suggested retail price.

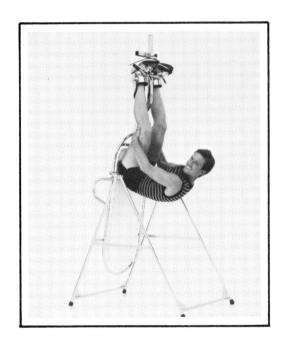

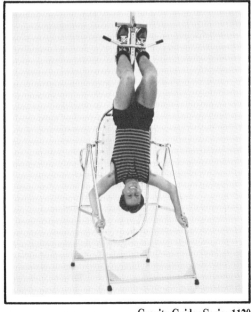

Gravity Guider Series 1120

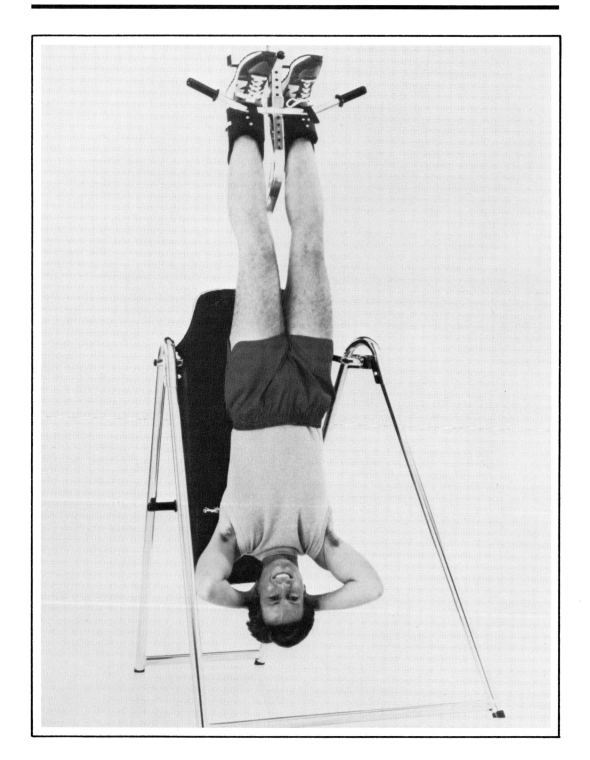

1121 Series A heavy-duty, 1 1/2'' chrome plated, steel tube ''A'' frame makes the 1121 Series durable and extra stable. The 1121 comes with a comfortable, black vinyl, uphostered bed that wipes clean after use. Height/weight adjustments for individuals 5' to 6'7'' and from 100 to 800 lbs. Folds for compact storage. $749.95

1130 Series This top-of-the-line model is the most complete inversion device available. Installs permanently (without holes) to floor and ceiling, and features a removable oscillation bed, an adjustable horizontal bar assist mechanism, and parallel dip bars. Made of 1 1/2'' chrome-plated tube steel, the unit is height/weight adjustable for individuals 5' to 6'6'' and from 100 to 500 lbs. Removable vinyl-coated, hand-roped canvas bed is for oscillation only. Stationary horizontal bar is for full inversion. Nice features on the unit are hand grips, which help with a variety of exercises, and an assist mechanism for chin-ups and other exercises. A Toggle Bar pivotal fitness bar attaches to the horizontal bar for upper body exercises. Price: $1,295.99

1150 Series For the budget minded, this unit comes with a black-matte finish and black nylon bed. Made of 1'' steel tube, the 1150 has a wide footprint for stability and a height/weight adjustment for individuals 5' to 6'6'' and from 100 to 300 lbs. Folds for storage. Price: $229.95

Accessories include: Inversion Boots (black finish) $59.95, (chrome finish) $84.95; Inversion Bar, $22.95; Xer-Sizer Bar, $69.95; Toggle Bar Pivot fitness bar, $89.95

◄ **Gravity Guider Series 1121**

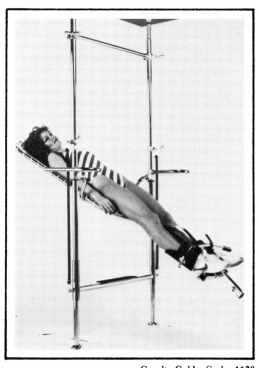

Gravity Guider Series 1130

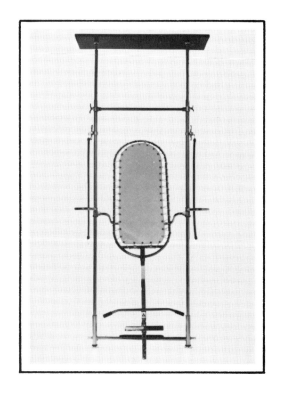

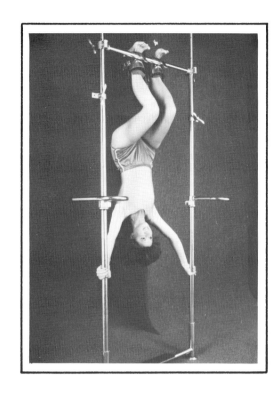

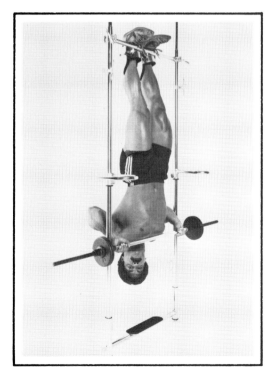

Huffy Sporting Goods

P.O. Box 07493
Milwaukee, Wisconsin 53207
1-800-558-5234, (414) 482-4240

   Huffy is the largest bicycle manufacturer in the world. The quality of its cycles is widely recognized. For example, the company supplied bicycles used in the 1984 Olympics. But Huffy also is fast becoming a leading manufacturer of home fitness equipment. And two of its products, the Workhorse and Body Ess, are totally new to the market. Call or write for brochures and the name of the nearest dealer.

Exercise cycles

Aerobic Fitness Cycle 500   Huffy's best cycle, this model features a twelve-pound chrome flywheel with nylon belt tension system, heavy-duty steel "H" frame construction, and a smooth free-wheeling hub. One exciting feature is a built-in "Pulse Data" unit with sensors in the handlebar that track pulse-rate, time, speed, and distance traveled. This compact bike has

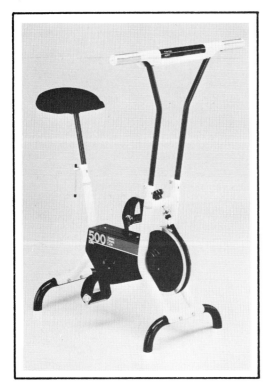

◄ Aerobic Fitness Cycle 500   Triathlon ►

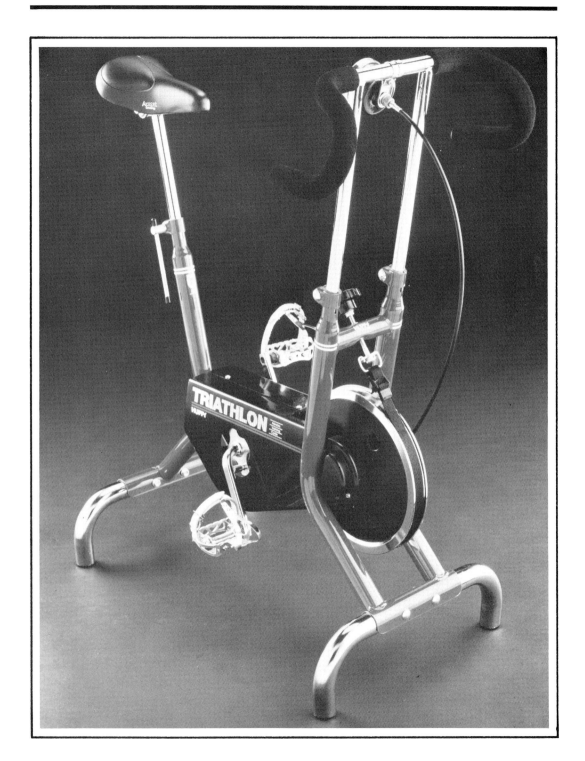

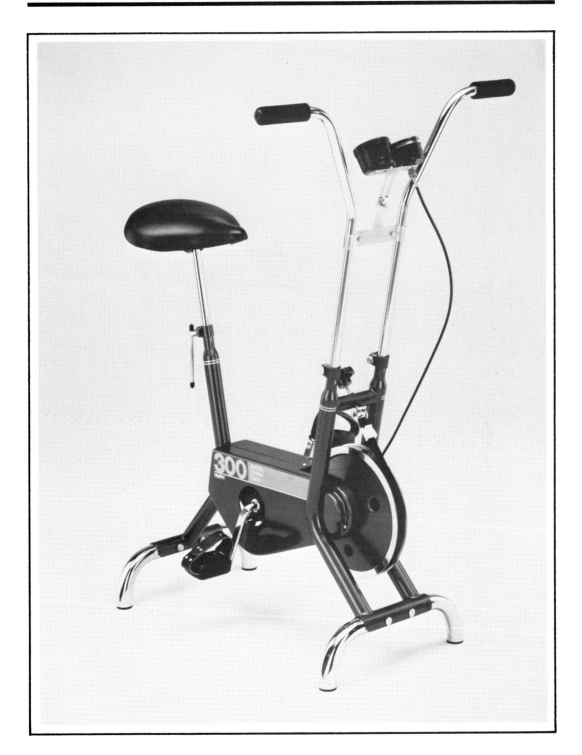

a low center of gravity, wide stabilizer bars, and adjustable contoured seat and handlebars. Color: artic white with black chain guards. Price: $290.00

Aerobic Fitness Cycles Five other cycles are available in this line. Aerobic Fitness Cycles 300 and 250 have nylon belt tension systems; weighted stirrup pedals; adjustable dual handlebars; contoured saddles with quick adjusts; heavy-duty steel "H" frames; chrome cast metal flywheels (on 300 and 250); enclosed chain guards; and speedometer, odometer, and timer. Colors: chrome and midnight blue (on 300);

metallic gray (on 250). UPS. Prices (300): $199.00; (250) $179.00

Lower-priced Aerobic Fitness Cycles 200, 150, and 100 feature steel "H" frames and clutch-type pivot brake/variable tension systems. All tension systems are fully enclosed. Colors: cinnamon (on 200); wine (on 150); and light beige (on 100). Prices: (200) $99.00; (150) $99.00; (100) $69.00

Triathalon A racy addition to Huffy's line, this bike features adjustable racing-style handlebars and saddle; chrome cast metal flywheel with nylon belt

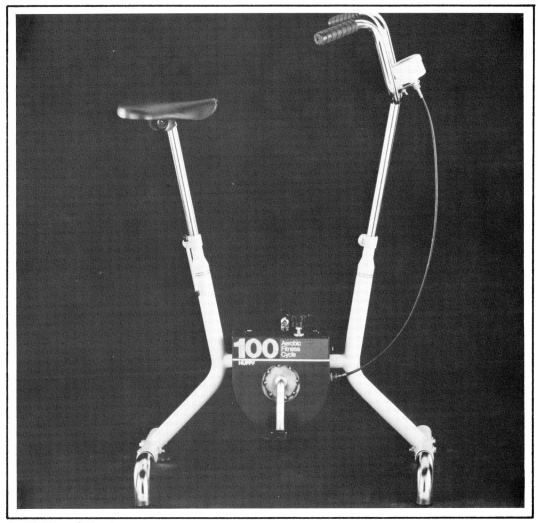

◄ Aerobic Fitness Cycles ▲

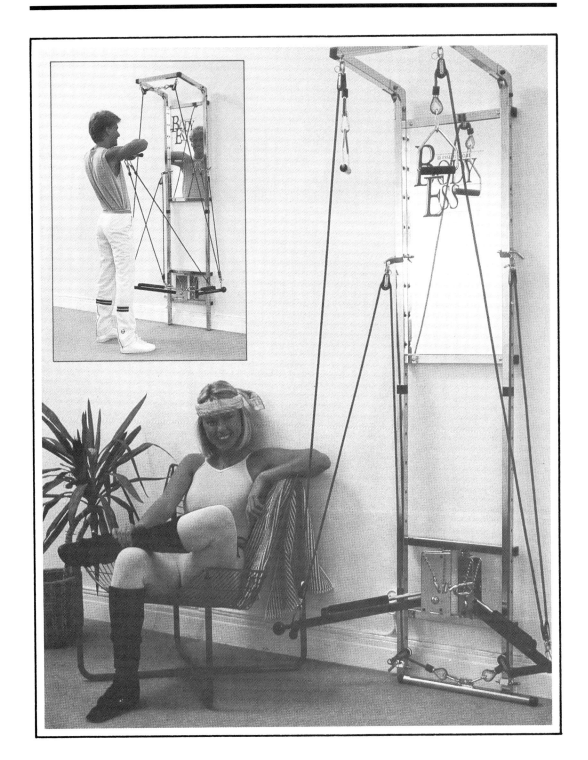

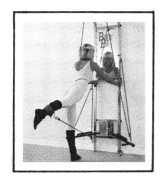

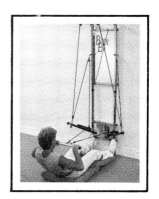

Body Ess —Huffy

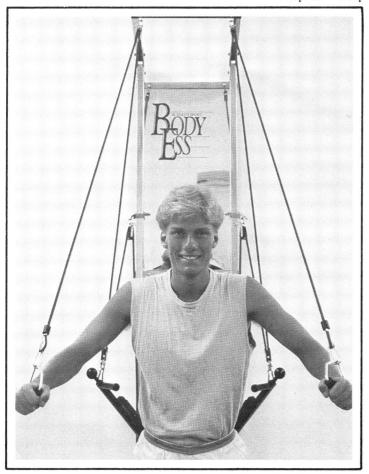

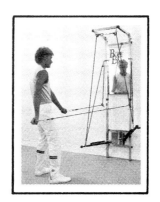

tension system; freewheeling hub; racing pedals with toe clips; and heavy-duty steel "H" frame. Comes with speedometer and odometer. Colors: Fiera red with black enclosed chain guard. Price: $229.00

Other exercise cycles   Huffy also makes several models with caliper tension systems and with roller tension systems. These bikes come in a variety of colors with color-coordinated seats and tires. All are made of heavy-duty steel frames with oval main tube construction. Price range: $69.00 to $129.00

Home gyms

Body Ess   Crafted in Sweden, Body Ess is the high-tech answer to resistance training. The system is capable of more than forty exercises designed to trim, tone, and shape. It relies on two air-compression pistons, called "power packs," that provide maximum resistance up to 120 kilograms (about 265 pounds) through a series of adjustable levers and pulleys. Each power pack provides a smooth, even range of resistance from six to seventy-two kilograms (about thirteen pounds to 159 pounds) for light, medium, and heavy resistance exercises. Wall-mounted, Body Ess requires only a few square feet of floor space, consisting of a steel tube frame, a crossbar, and two power packs. Also provided are two hand pulleys, a bar exerciser, and nylon rope. Price: $249.00

Rowers

Workhorse   A cross between a rower and a fun ride, the Workhorse gives a full-body aerobic workout. The user sits on a comfortable vinyl saddle and pushes with feet while pulling with hands. A curling exercise is also possible by pulling the handle underhanded. With each pull, a fully enclosed mechanism gives an up and down ride motion. The Workhorse has twenty-six resistance settings and adjustable handle and footrest. A square steel tube base with four supports provides strength and stability. The seating unit is made of high impact plastic. Color: black with red trim. Price: $199.00

Deluxe Rowing System (model 7010)   A single beam raised two degrees and concave, ball bearing seat rollers give this rower a very smooth ride. Dual hydraulic pistons are adjustable to three tension positions and independent arms have a 360-degree rowing arc and ball bearing pivots. The system features a well-padded seat and independently angled foot pedals with fastening straps. The main frame is made of aluminum. Color: black, aluminum. Price: $199.00

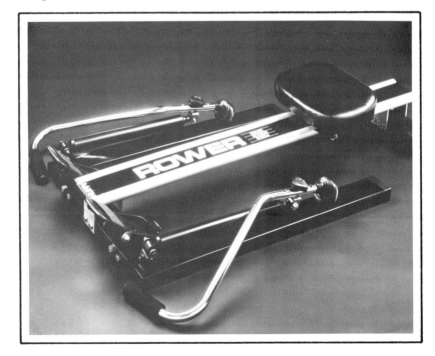

Workhorse ▶

◀ Deluxe Rowing System

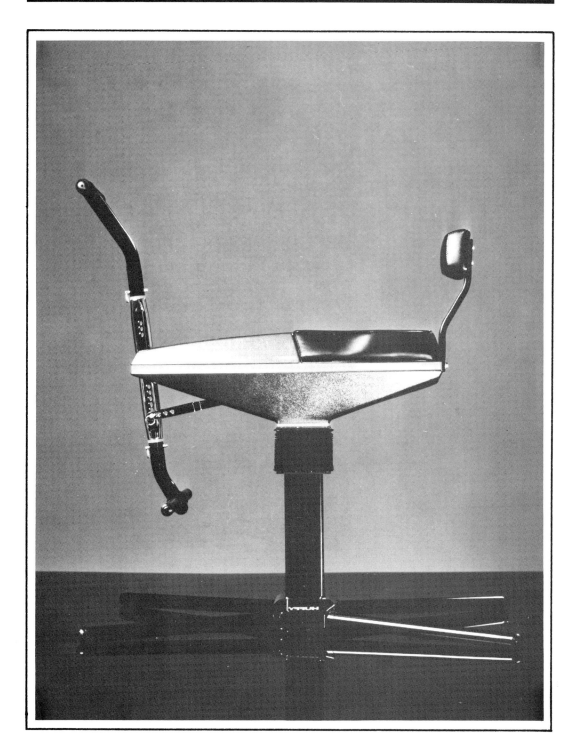

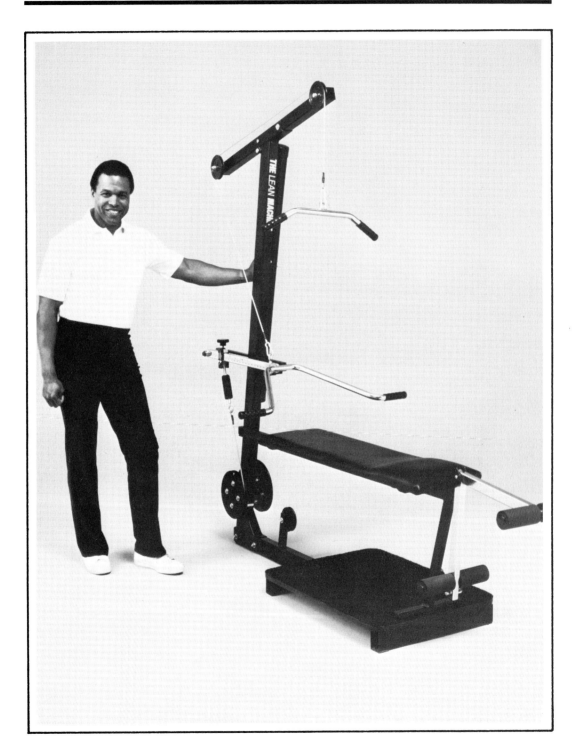

The Lean Machine Inc.

7245 S. Harl
Tempe, Arizona 85283
1-800-821-7143, 264-7009 (in Arizona)

A division of Inertia Dynamics Corporation, this innovative young company has built a multi-million dollar success on a single product: the Lean Machine. Endorsed by Gale Sayers, All-American and member of the Professional Football Hall of Fame, this machine is remarkably versatile and easy to use. The company offers a lifetime warranty on all parts and workmanship, and a thirty-day money back guarantee on deliveries. The Lean Machine is available direct from the manufacturer, and a new model is available in some retail outlets. On direct orders, the company accepts major credit cards and CODs (with down payment).

Home gyms

The Lean Machine A resistance system that relies on cams, pulleys, and levers makes this multi-gym unique. Two concealed thirty-inch counterforce springs provide resistance up to 200 pounds at the pressing station and 250 pounds at the pulley station. An optional Heavy Duty Resistance package increases press station resistance to 280 pounds and

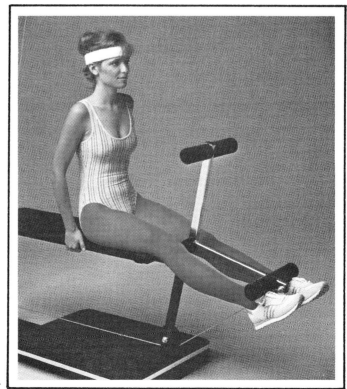

◀ The Lean Machine ▶

pulley to 350 pounds. A special selector scale allows infinite tension settings. As pressure is exerted, a cam action equalizes resistance throughout the entire range of movement.

Capable of forty-five exercises, this free-standing machine offers a pressing station, upper and lower pullies, a padded leg extension/leg curl station, and a padded bench which can be removed or inclined for sit-ups. Removing the bench leaves a carpeted platform, from which a variety of standing and kneeling exercises may be performed. Total workout area is approximately three and one-half by seven feet.

Standard equipment includes three chrome-plated exercise bars, chrome leg fixture, heavy-duty nylon-coated cables, sturdy bearing pulley and cam assemblies. The machine is constructed of heavy-gauge steel tube frame. LWH: 92″ × 24″ × 82½″. Shipping weight: 187 lbs. Price: $695.00 plus $60.00 shipping; (COD) $395.00 in advance, then $300.00, plus shipping, and COD charges in cash or certified check on delivery.

The Lean Machine Pro This new model has a sleek, sculptured look and the same basic features of the original model. It is sold through a growing number of retail outlets. Price: $695.00

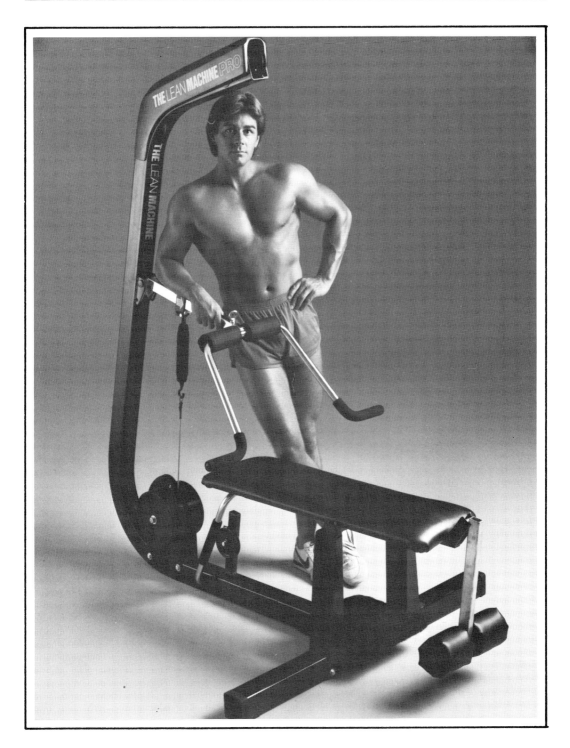

Marcy Fitness Products

2801 West Mission Road
Alhambra, California 91803
(213) 570-1222

Marcy home fitness equipment is among the best available. The company, founded in 1946, is an innovator with long experience in design and manufacture of quality training equipment.

Marcy is found in the White House, and in the homes of Clint Eastwood, Cheryl Tiegs, Sylvester Stallone, and many other celebrities. More importantly, it is widely available for installation in your home. Marcy home equipment can be found almost anywhere, and you can expand equipment as your budget allows.

Home gyms

EM-1 Marcy's hottest seller is one of the most complete home gyms available. Wall-mounted or free-standing (optional), the unit features fourteen stations to exercise all muscle groups. The EM-1 comes with a 200-pound black, captured weight stack (optional 120-pound add-on kit), and the user can switch weights to various stations with a simple turn of a lever. The EM-1 has a ten-position lifting arm, lat bar, incline bench with leg extension/leg curl assembly, and an arm curl with rowing station. The unit features aluminum I-beam construction. Price: $650.00

Bodybar Fitness Center An incredible duo, the fitness center includes Bodybar 2000 and Body Toner, which attaches to make the center free-standing. Both units feature sturdy steel construction with captured cast iron weights available in black.

Bodybar 2000 Comes with 100-pound weight stack in ten-pound increments (optional kit gives 180-pound total resistance). Bodybar has an eight-position lifting arm with self-locking pins. A versatile pulley system offers two positions, single and double cable handles, and padded ankle strap. A workout bench/leg developer has raised knee padding for leg extensions, four-inch padding, and two-inch steel rollers. The padded bench detaches for abdominal exercises. The Power Bar accessory accomodates 120-pound barbell plates. Other accessories include a latissimus bar for upper body development and a leg press bar that attaches to the Bodybar carriage. The unit may be wall-mounted or free-standing with support bar accessory. Price: $299.00 (100 lb. stack); $399.00 (180 lb. stack).

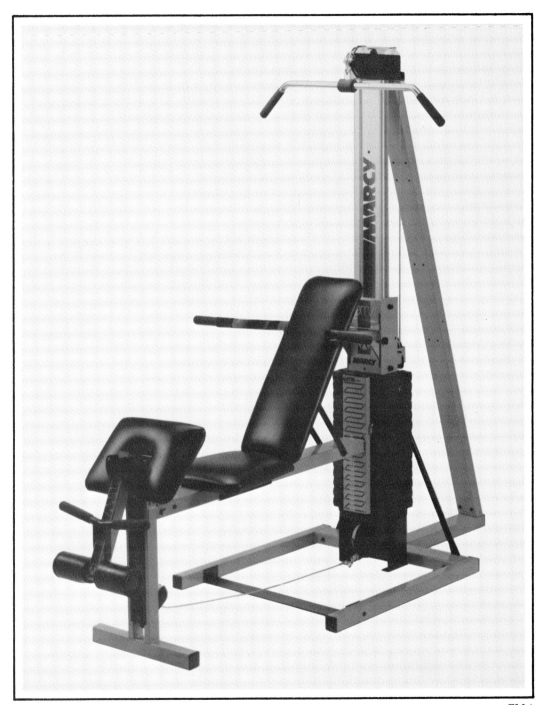

EM-1

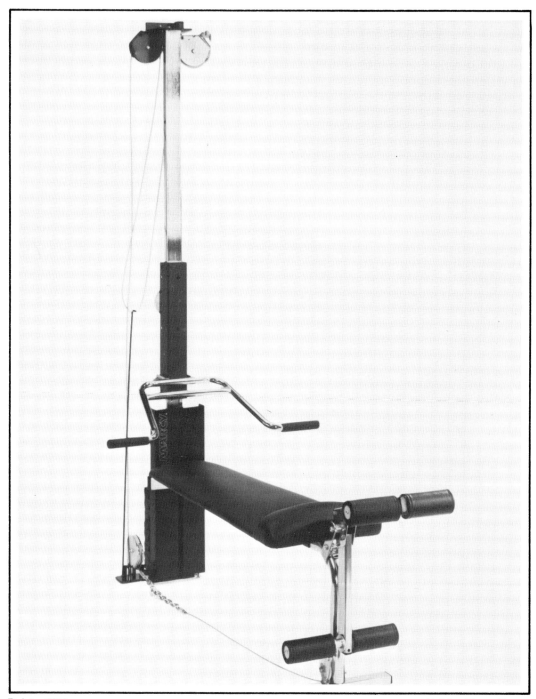

Bodybar 2000

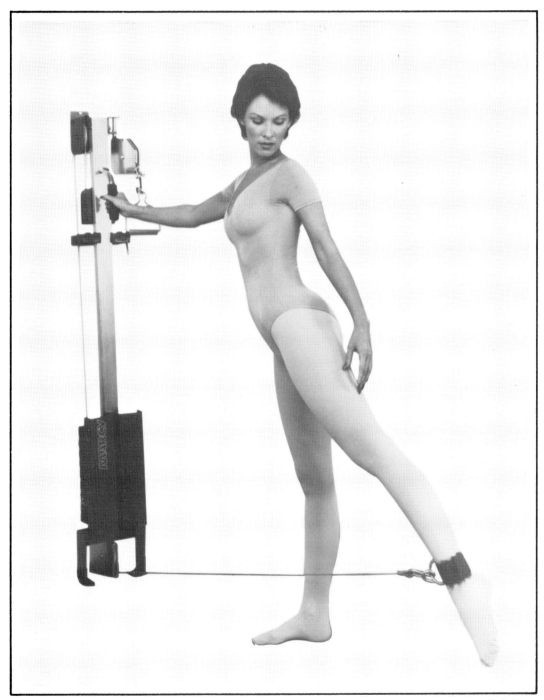

Body Toner

Body Toner   This unit has a single weight stack: fifty pounds in five-pound increments, or 100 pounds in ten-pound increments. It features two pulleys, one at shoulder height and one at floor level, for a variety of barbell-pulley type exercises. Body Toner also can be free-standing with optional accessory ($100.00). LWH: 12″ × 6″ × 67″. Price: $250.00 (50 lb. stack).

Master Gym Series   The modular design with two, three, or four stations allows equipment selection based on space or budget. All equipment is constructed with heavy-duty steel. The unit is free-standing. Each station has a captured weight stack. Cast iron weights are available in black lacquer (standard) or chrome (optional). The finish is available in silver vein (standard) and chrome (optional). Each unit has nylon coated cables and maintenance-free bearings on all moving parts.

The following stations are included in the series.

MACH 1 Press Station   Rugged construction with 220-pound (optional 260-pound) weight stacks. This station requires less than one square foot of floor space. The unit performs dozens of barbell exercises and features an adjustable lifting arm with eight starting heights. It has been lab tested for a million-plus repetitions, and easily expands with optional accessories (power bar, leg press, low bench).

Quad Pulley   The versatile Quad-Pulley design allows all major dumbbell and pulley exercises. Dual weight stacks (fifty-pound or 100-pound each) are equipped with steel weight guards. Four pulleys with two handles each at shoulder and floor heights permit independent action for arms and legs. The unit also includes hand grips and ankle straps for leg exercises.

Latissimus Machine   A popular basic, the lat machine provides a range of exercises for the upper body. The unit features an extra-wide (fifty-inch) pull-down bar and 180-pound weight stack that slides on a 2½″ wide steel column.

Abdominal Board   (included with lat station) features durable upholstery, heel rest, and padded ankle rollers with hand supports for leg raisers.

Optional Stations in Master Gym Series include:

Leg Station   The unit features a full-length padded table for leg curls and extensions, and comes with 120-pound weight stacks. The unit attaches to the Master Gym frame.

Hip Flexion Station   A great add-on, this offers padded back and arm supports for lower abdominal conditioning. It is adjustable for height, and attaches to the Master Gym frame.

Base prices for Master Gym   2-Station Gym: includes Mach 1, lat pull, workout bench and abdominal board. Requires 3′ × 12′ in use. $1,495.00
3-Station Gym: includes 2-station plus quad pull. Requires 8′ × 12′ in use. $1,995.00
4-Station Gym: includes 3-station plus leg extension, or hip flexion unit. Requires up to 12′ × 12′ in use. $2,250.00 (including Hip Flexion) to $2,650.00 (including leg extension)

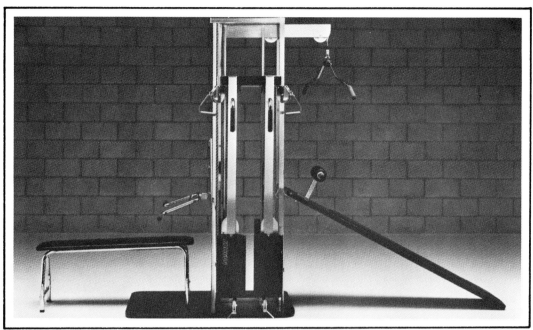

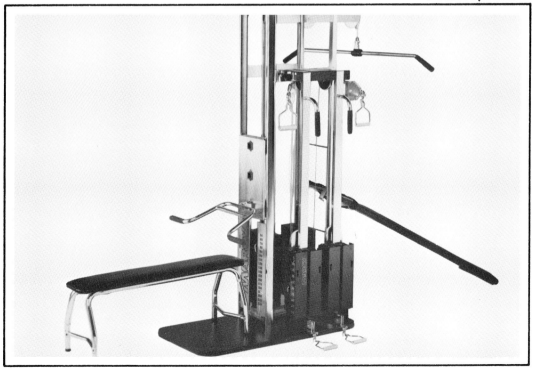

Treadmills

Pacesetter Treadmill This instrument features an inclined running surface with three elevation settings for fast, medium, or slow paces. The durable, shock absorbing running surface is designed for years of wear. The unit has eighteen 2″-diameter rollers with self-lubricating bearings and 4″-diameter flanged end rollers that help keep belt centered. LWH: 46″ × 24″ × 49″. Price: $500.00

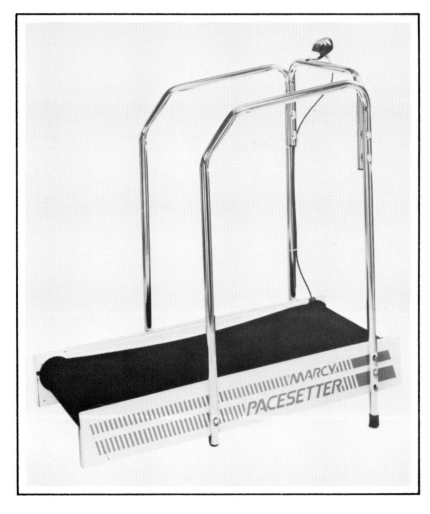

**Pacesetter Treadmill
—Marcy Fitness Products**

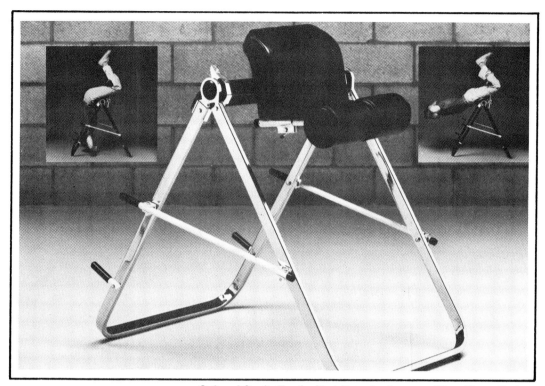

Orthopod Gravity Traction/Back Extension System —Marcy Fitness Products

Inversion boards

Orthopod Gravity Traction/Back Extension System Turning gravity to your back's advantage, this station is ideal for back hyperextensions, abdominal exercises, and spinal column decompression. It is easily mounted, and has comfortable padded pelvic and leg supports that pivot on 2¼" bearings. It is constructed of heavy-gauge tube steel. LWH: 44" × 30" × 38". Price: $330.00

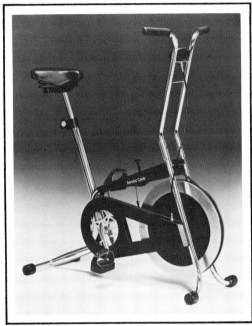

Avita 400 Aerobic Cycle ▲

▼ Avita 450 Professional Ergometer ▶

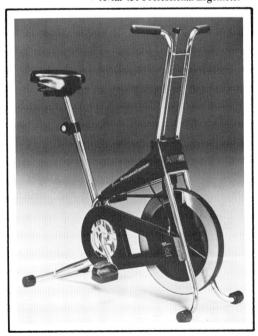

M & R Industries
9215 151st. Ave. Northeast
Redmond, Washington 98052
1-800-222-9995, (206) 885-1010

Maker of the "Avita" line of exercise equipment, M & R builds institutional quality into its products at affordable prices. Call for free brochures or a list of dealers in your area.

Exercise cycles

Avita 400 Aerobic Cycle   This bike features a forty-five-pound cast iron flywheel that keeps turning even through "dead" parts of the pedal stroke. Resistance is provided by a nylon strap; a console-mounted lever provides infinite tension adjustment. The frame is made of heavy-gauge steel with chrome plating. The 400 has a smooth operating ball bearing crank and pedals. Pedals come with adjustable toe straps. The 400 also comes with speedometer and resettable odometer. Colors: black, chrome. LWH: 38″ × 19″ × 42″. Weight: 76 lbs. One year warranty on parts, materials, and workmanship. Price: $325.00

Avita 450 Professional Ergometer   This machine has the same basic design and construction as the Avita 400 with a few important extras. Resistance is provided by caliper-type, disc brakes with high-density felt pads. Resistance control, which is mounted near the handgrips, permits load levels from free-wheeling to 400 watts. Instrumentation in the console includes watt-meter, pedal RPM indicator, odometer, and sixty-minute timer. The flywheel has a special, no-mar tire that doubles as transportation roller. Weight: 78 lbs. Price: $475.00

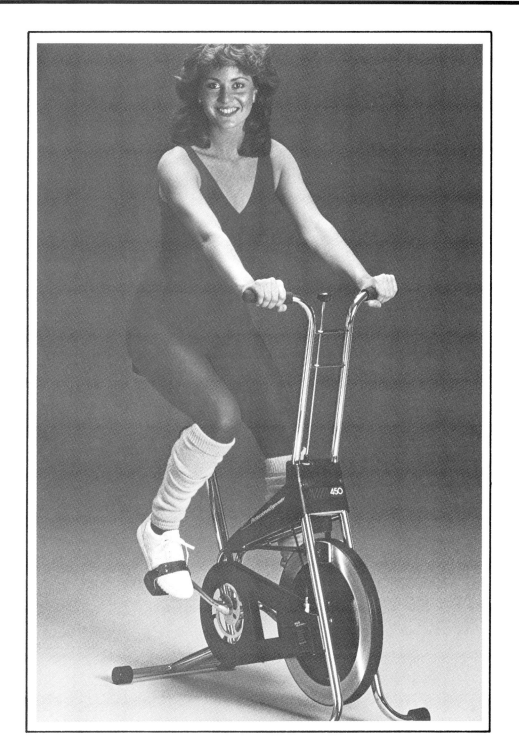

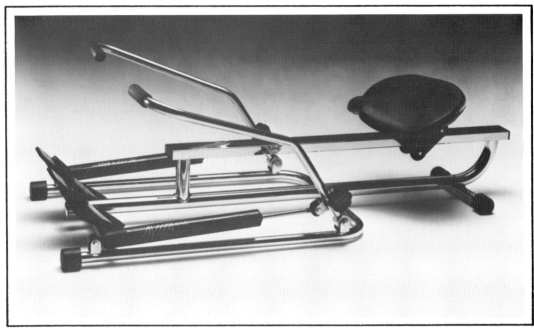

Avita 850 Aerobic Rower ▲

▼ Avita 950 Professional Rower ▶

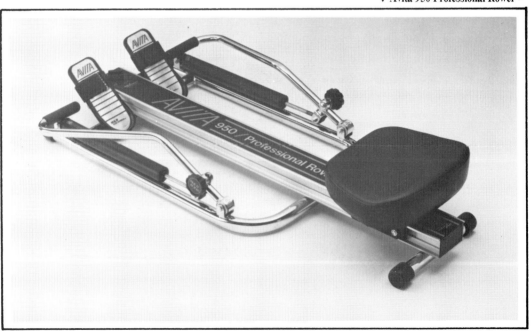

Rowers

Avita 850 Aerobic Rower A sturdy, one-piece steel frame prevents the 850 from walking while you're rowing. A contoured, cushioned seat rides on nylon rollers on a chromed steel track. A pouch of gas that expands and contracts in twin cylinders complements the hydraulic action of oil, providing resistance without "squishiness." Steel oar arms turn on sealed ball bearing pivots. Cast aluminum swivel footplates with wide straps move independently as you row. LWH: 54″ × 30″ × 13″. Weight: 47 lbs. Price: $330.00

Avita 950 Professional Rower Although it has the same basic construction of the 850 Rower, the 950 features several top quality improvements and accessories. A deluxe cushioned seat glides on ball bearing rollers on an internal track. A cast aluminum center rail provides strength and a smooth ride. The 950 includes a sixty-minute timer. Accessories include a bench board that allows the 950 to stand on end, making possible bench press, squats, curls, and other exercises; a seat lock assembly that facilitates sit-ups and backward seated exercises; swivel hand grips (also fit 850); and a deluxe seat cover. LWH: 49″ × 30″ × 9½″. Weight: 41 lbs. Price: (950 Rower) $350.00; (950XL version, which has an aluminum rail that is 6″ longer) $450.00; (seat lock) $19.95; (deluxe seat cover) $13.95; (swivel grips) $10.95

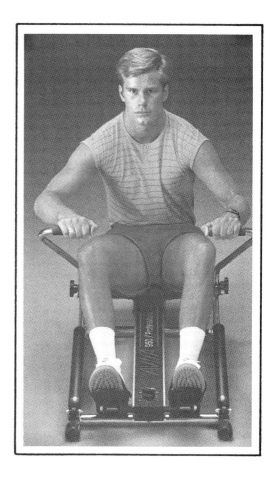

Treadmills

Avita 300 Manual Treadmill A fingertip pace control lets you start and end your run gradually. Pacing brake governs speed from one-half to twenty-five mph. The endless rubber belt with waffle tread rolls over sound-deadening aluminum rollers for smooth, quiet operation. The running surface is 16″ × 40″. Variable incline adjustment elevates the grade from 2% to 14%. A speedometer/tripometer indicates speed and distance. A fold-down handrail allows for storage on end. The unit rolls on casters, and its body is constructed of heavy-duty steel frame. LWH: 46½″ × 25½″ × 48″ (12″ high with folded handrail). Weight: 133 lbs. Color: metallic gray, chrome. Price: $699.00

Avita 350 Electric Treadmill This unit features a tough, 1½ hp motor, six-pound, dynamically balanced flywheel, and cog-belt drive for maintenance-free power on demand. Speed range is infinitely adjustable at the fingertip console from zero to ten mph. Belt speed responds gradually to prevent jerks and stops. The console also has a sixty-minute timer.

The running surface measures 50″ × 15″, and is made of antistatic, PVC/polyester, cord-backed belt for quiet, low friction operation. Rubber coated, tapered-end rollers have sealed ball bearings for long life. The 350's frame is made of sturdy anodized aluminum with chromed front rail. The motor runs on standard household current. Weight: 152 lbs. LWH: 61″ × 21¾″ × 51″. Price: $1,200.00

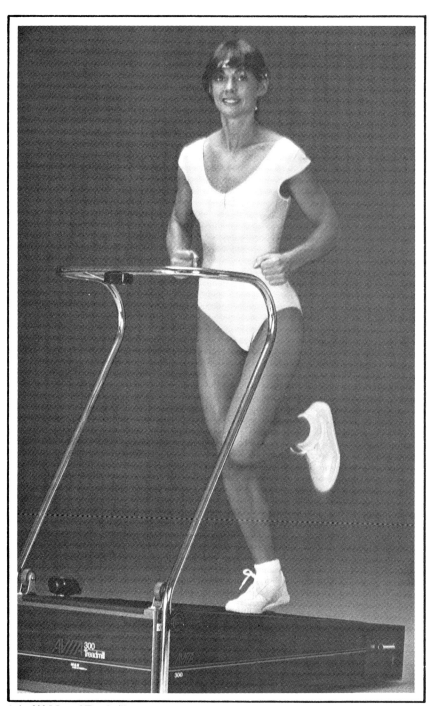

Avita 300 Manual Treadmill

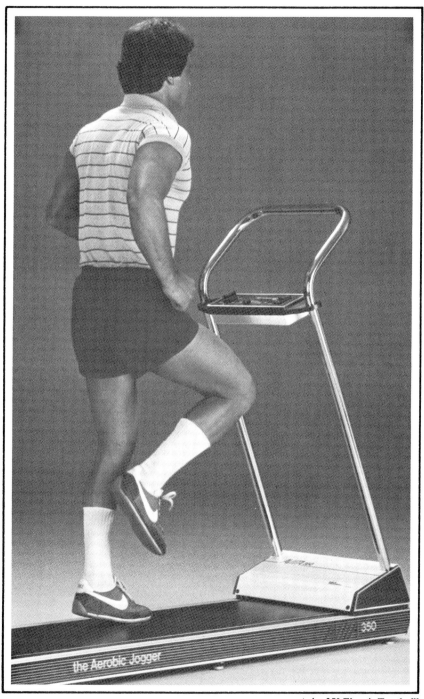

Avita 350 Electric Treadmill

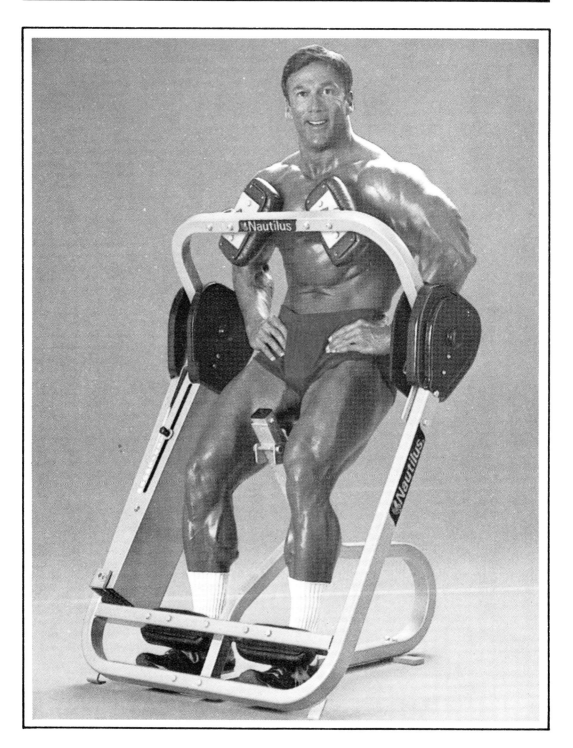

Nautilus for the Home

P.O. Box 1119
Lake Helen, Florida 32744
1-800-321-3551, (904) 228-2884 (in Florida)

Nautilus equipment has revolutionized fitness training for college and professional athletes, and now the company is tackling the home fitness market. Patterning its home equipment after its commercial units, Nautilus now sells two single-function machines: one for abdominal exercise and one for the lower back.

Nautilus equipment is available direct from the manufacturer, as well as from some retailers and catalog operations. On direct orders, the company accepts major credit cards, personal checks, and money orders. Machines come with a thirty-day unconditional money-back guarantee.

Home gyms

Abdominal Machine   This machine isolates and exercises the abdominal muscles. In this, it is an improvement over sit-ups and leg raisers, which tend to concentrate on the hip flexor muscles. The exercise is performed from a seated position by pushing a padded movement arm forward and down, then pulling slowly back and up to the start position. A special Nautilus cam (which resembles a deep sea nautilus shell) automatically varies the amount of resistance through the entire range of movement. Resistance is supplied by elastic cords that are housed inside the machine. As strength improves, nine tension settings from mild to strenuous permit gradually increased resistance. The unit is constructed of heavy-duty tube steel frame. All contact surfaces are cushioned with high-density foam and covered with Naugahyde. Easy assembly. LWH: 38″ X 35½″ X 48″. Weight: 150 lbs. Price: $485.00 plus $55.00 shipping.

Lower Back Machine   Designed to strengthen the long muscles of the back, this is the home version of a similar machine designed for commercial and medical use. The exercise begins in a bent, standing position with feet on an adjustable foot pad and buttocks resting against an inclined pad. A belt straps across the hips. The exercise is performed by pushing a padded movement arm back into a standing, inclined position, then pulling slowly forward into the start position. This machine features the same construction, easy assembly (eight bolts to tighten), and resistance principle (with nine tension levels) as the Abdominal Machine. LWH: 51″ X 35″ X 54″. Weight: 150 lbs. Price: $485.00 plus $55.00 shipping.

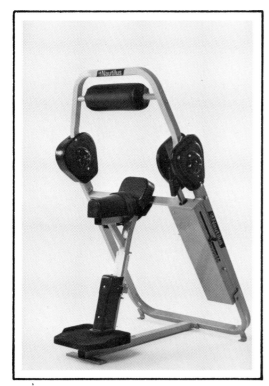

◄ **Abdominal Machine**   ▲ **Lower Back Machine**

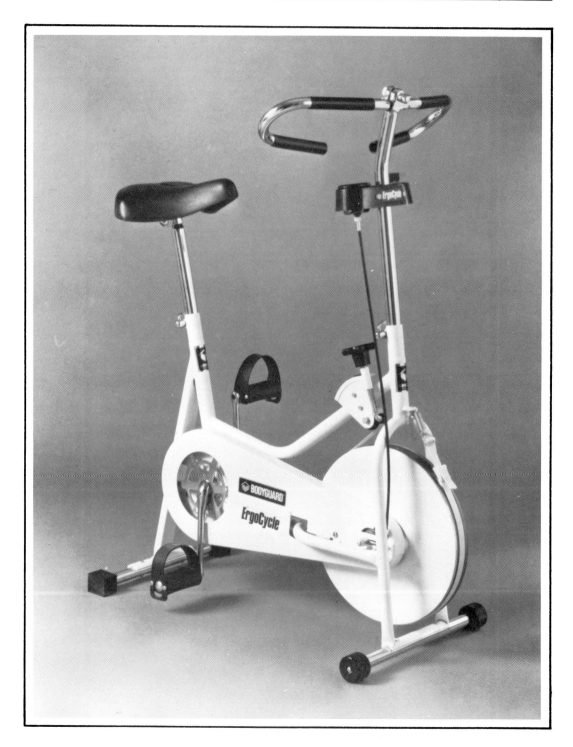

J. Oglaend Inc.
40 Radio Circle
Mt. Kisco, NY 10549-0096
1-800-828-1186, (914) 666-2272

This is the United States headquarters for Bodyguard products, which are built by Jonas Oglaend of Norway, Scandinavia's largest bicycle manufacturer. Excellent quality and reliability is built into each product. Call for brochures and the name of your nearest dealer.

Exercise cycles

Bodyguard 955 This bike features a low center of gravity and a solid, 30 lb. flywheel with Herculon weave friction resistance strap. Built of heavy-duty tube steel, the bike features an enclosed chain drive, hardened steel crank, and comfortable pedals. The steel frame has a lifetime warranty. The bike also has quick-release seat and handlebar adjustments. Instruments include a unique, built-in calibration mechanism for the workload scale, which helps to accurately measure pedaling load in watts and Newton-meters. Other instruments include speedometer/odometer and timer. The 955 requires 21" x 38" floor space. Weight: 70 lbs. LWH: 33"x16"x41" (seat height ranges from 30" to 41"). Color: white enamel. Price: $395.00

Bodyguard 957 Basically the same quality materials and workmanship as the 955, this cycle features racing handlebars and seat, as well as pedals with toe clips and straps. Weight: 60 lbs. LWH: 33"x16"x41" (seat height ranges from 30" to 41". Color: white enamel. Price: $425.00

◀ **Bodyguard 955**　　　▼ **Bodyguard 957**

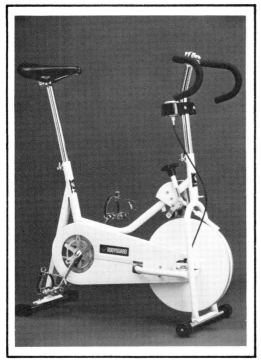

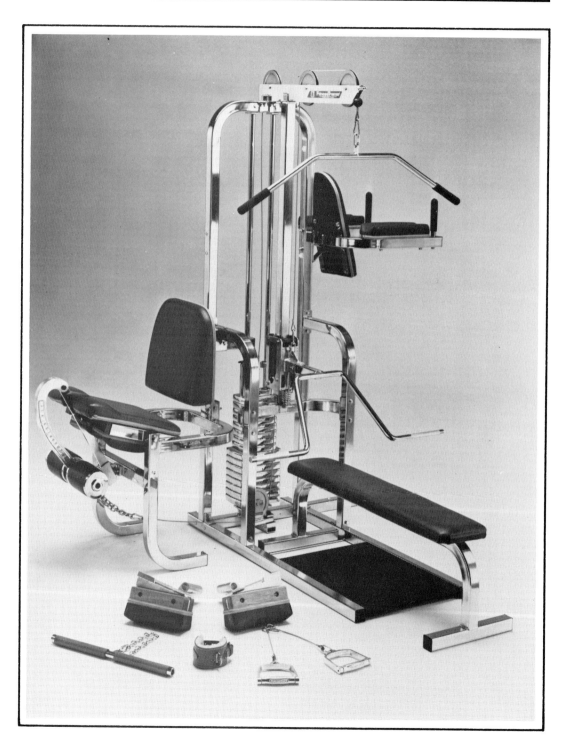

Paramount Fitness Equipment
6450 E. Bandini Blvd.
Los Angeles, California 90040
(213) 721-3644

Paramount builds professional quality into its home gyms at a reasonable price. Call for free brochures or for the dealer nearest you.

Home gyms

FitnessMate This is a superbly crafted, free-standing gym capable of exercising all muscle groups. Constructed of two-inch tube steel with nickel-chrome plating, the unit comes with 170-pound captured weight stack in ten-pound increments (fifteen-pound increments optional); ball-bearing pulleys at the top and bottom; aircraft quality cables; and Naugahyde covered, padded bench with padded leg extension/leg curl assembly. Standard equipment includes lat and bench press bars, pulley bar, and padded ankle strap. The unit fits into less than a thirty-square-foot workout area. Weights come in black or chrome (optional); 230-pound stack also available. Shipping weight: 430–490 lbs. Price range: $1,395.00 to $1,895.00

FitnessTrainer II This unit has a removable bench with padded platform underneath for standing and kneeling exercises. Options include seated leg extension/leg curl station, padded leg press/squat device that attaches to press bar, padded vertical knee raise station, sit-up board with foot strap and adjustable rack, and Roman bench (for back raisers) with adjustable roller pads. The unit requires less than a sixty-square-foot workout area. Shipping weight: 629 to 669 lbs. Price: (basic unit) $2,700.00

FitnessTrainer I This deluxe model has the same free-standing construction of FitnessTrainer II with two weight stacks. Chest press, shoulder press, leg press, and squat exercises have 210-pound stack (310-pound optional); leg extension/leg curl, low and high pulley exercises have 105-pound stack (155-pound optional). Other options and prices are the same as FitnessTrainer II. The unit requires less than a sixty-square-foot workout area. Weight: 820 lbs. Price: (basic unit) $3,200.00

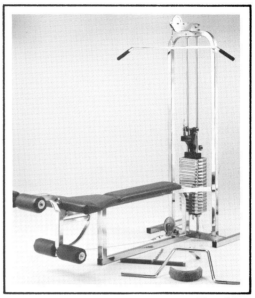

FitnessMate

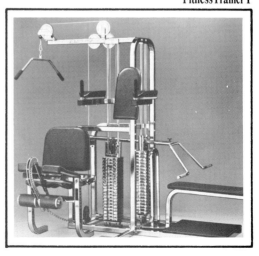

FitnessTrainer I

Precor USA

9449 151st Ave. Northeast
Redmond, Washington 98052
(206) 881-8982

Precor is earning a reputation as the manufacturer of some of most beautifully designed home fitness equipment. But the company also is known for the excellent quality and durability of its products. It is difficult to go wrong buying from this manufacturer. Call or write for brochures and Precor dealers nearest you.

Exercise cycles

820e Electronic Bicycle This precision cycle has microprocessor electronics for accurate controls and feedback. The electronic module features a micro-adjust tension knob that moves through a regulated scale, which allows users to accurately set and reset workload levels. The electronic display (powered by a nine-volt battery) shows elapsed time, pedal rpm, and distance.

Power is transferred to the 25 lb. flywheel through a v-belt drive system, giving the 820e an exceptionally quiet, smooth ride. This design eliminates chain and freewheel noise, and the mess from chain lubrication.

The 820e is made of anodized aircraft aluminum and precision molded parts, which give it a sleek profile. Handlebars have four position settings and padded grips. Seat is adjustable from 31″ to 39″. Required floor space is 16″x25 1/2″. Height at handlebars is 42″. Color: black, aluminum. Price: $500.00

Precor 820 Electronic Bicycle ▶

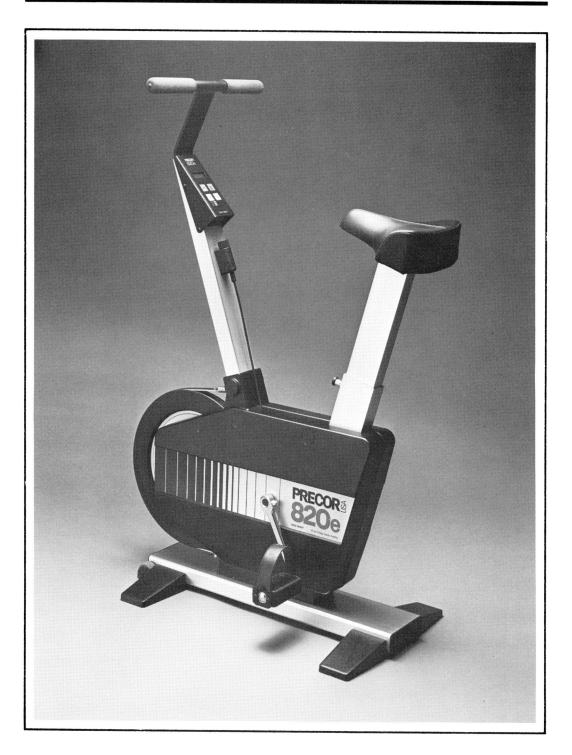

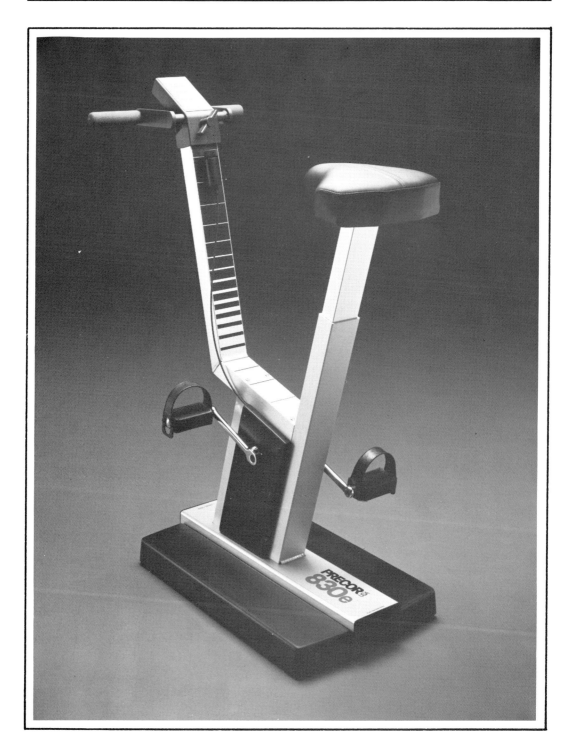

830e Bicycle Ergometer A horizonatally mounted, 25 lb. flywheel gives the 830e a very smooth, quiet ride. It uses direct drive gearing, which eliminates messy and noisy chains. The cycle's bearings are completely sealed and maintenance free.

A nine-volt battery powers a microprocessor that gives readouts on elapsed time, pedaling rpm, distance, work rate (in calories per minute), and total calorie expenditure. The control panel is moisture proof and offers fingertip mode selection.

A nice feature is the padded handgrips, which rotate in a full circle. The padded seat also is adjustable from 31'' to 39''. The body is made of extruded anodized aluminum and precision molded 4.B.S. plastic. Color: black, aluminum. Required floor space is 16'' × 25½''. Weight: 60 lbs. Price: $800.00

Rowers

600 Single Piston Rowing Machine A lightweight, compact rower that requires only 15''x48'' floor space. Weighing only 23 lbs., it is easily moved and stored vertically. The rower features an anodized aluminum rail, and a contoured, padded seat with a ball bearing roller carriage. Although it has a single piston, the unit's new valving system for the hydraulic cylinders offers a load range of five to 175 lbs. Other features include rotating handgrips, and pivoting footplates with adjustable straps. Colors: black, aluminum. Price: $195.00

◄ **Precor 830e Bicycle Ergometer**

▼ **Precor 600 Single Piston Rowing Machine**

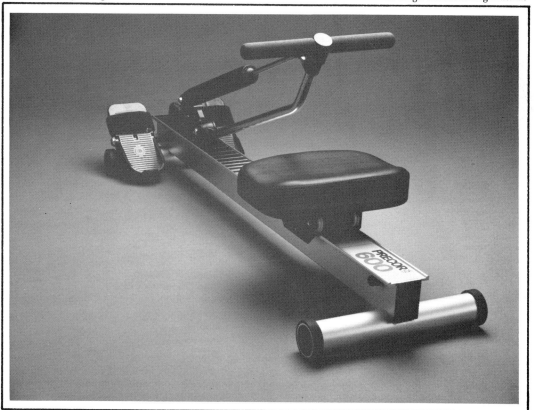

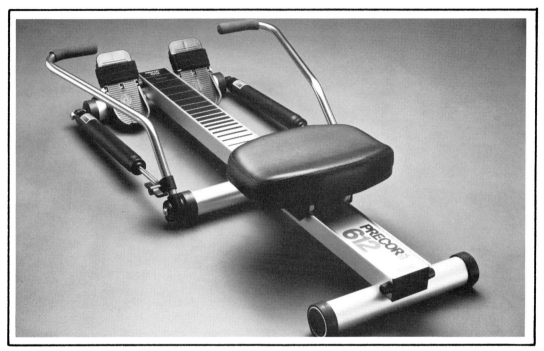

Precor 612 Dual Piston Rowing Machine

612 Dual Piston Rowing Machine This lightweight machine is made of sturdy stainless steel welded into a box beam frame. Rowing arms are made of sturdy, chrome plated steel. Dual, oil filled, hydraulic cylinders feature the latest in engineering design with a new valving system that gives smooth, quiet action. The unit offers an infinitely adjustable load range from 10 to 300 lbs. Other features include pivoting footplates with adjustable straps, ball bearing seat carriage, and vertical storage. Weight: 30 lbs. Required floor space: 30" × 52". Color: black, aluminum. Price: $285.00

620e Dual Piston Professional Rowing Machine This model offers many of the features found on the 612 rower, with an extra long, anodized aluminum frame, strengthening stabilizer bars and microprocessor controlled electronics, which display time, strokes per minute, and total strokes. This rower is built for the strongest, most enthusiastic oarsmen. The oversized, oil-filled hydraulic cylinders have a specially designed valving system for smooth, quiet action. The unit offers an infinitely adjustable load range from 10 to 300 lbs. Required floor space: 32" × 52". Weight: 44 lbs. Stores vertically. Color: black, aluminum. Price: $425.00

630e Rowing Ergometer This is the first true rowing ergometer designed for home use. Microprocessor controlled electronics give accurate readings of elapsed time, stroke rate, total strokes, work rate (in calories per minute), and total caloric expenditure. With many of the same quality features found on the 612 and 620e rowers, this is another model built for active use. For example, the frame is able to accomodate any size user. Required floor space: 30"x51". Weight: 43 lbs. Stores vertically. Color: black, aluminum. Price: $600.00

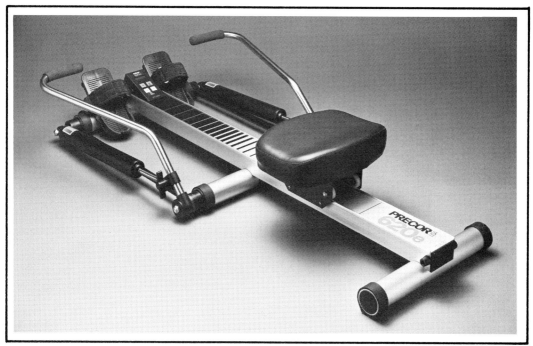

Precor 620e Dual Piston Professional Rowing Machine ▲   ▼ Precor 630e Rowing Ergometer

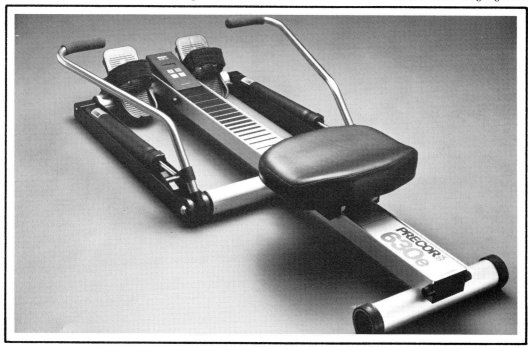

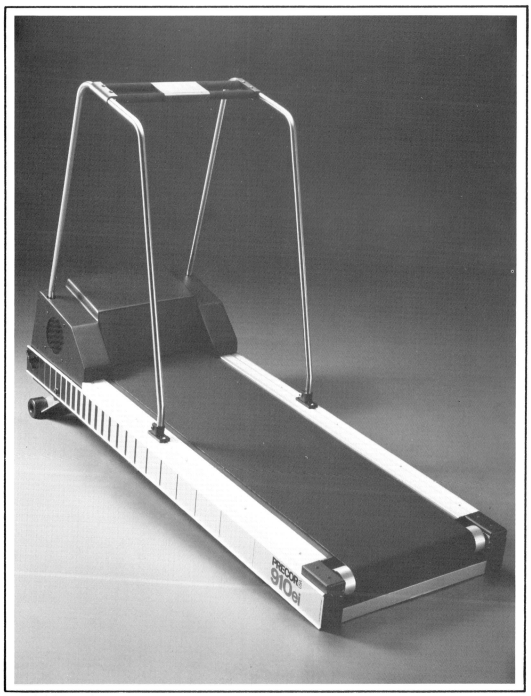

Precor 910ei Treadmill

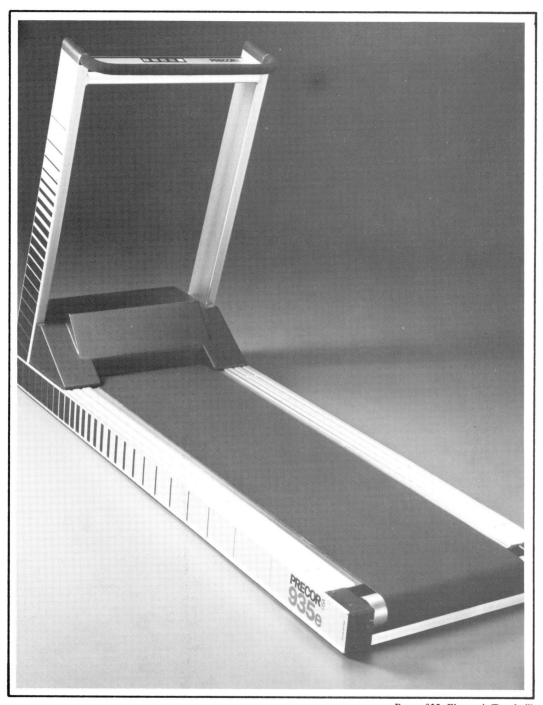

Precor 935e Electronic Treadmill

Treadmills

910e Treadmill This motorized treadmills features a 1 hp DC motor with variable speed control from one to eight mph, adjustable to each tenth mph. A nice feature of the specially regulated motor is the elimination of momentary surges and stalls from each footplant. A microcomputer controlled, fingertip key pad puts the user in direct control of pace, stopping and starting. A digital display shows total elapsed time, speed, and total mileage. The unit uses a light strobe to accurately measure speed and distance.

The 910e is made of anodized aluminum for durability without excessive weight, and rollers utilize maintenance-free sealed ball bearings. The running belt is a special non-strech, elastomer material. Running surface: 54"x17". LWH: 69"x26"x43". Required floor space: 26"x69". Weight: 145 lbs. Price: $2,200.00

910ei Treadmill Precor's most popular treadmill. Basically the same as the 910e, this model includes a gas spring-assisted arm that inclines the running bed to simulate hills, with grade settings from zero to 15 percent. LWH: 72"x26"x43". Weight: 155 lbs. Price: $2,400.00

935e Electronic Treadmill One of the finest treadmills made today, the 935e features all-new, microprocessor controlled electronics that measure time, speed, distance, calories per minute, and total caloric expenditure. Body weight and speed are set by the user with simple fingertip controls, and the 935e does the rest.

The treadmill also uses sophisticated technology to "read" each footplant, and it automatically adjusts belt speed to minimize "sticking" and "jerking," which are common to most treadmills. An elastomer running belt and special, low-friction bed design make for smooth, accurate footplants at any pace. The 935e features a 1 hp (DC) motor with variable speed control from one to ten mph, adjustable to each tenth mph. Made of anodized aluminum, with sealed, maintenance-free, ball bearing rollers, the 935e is built for lasting function, strength and durability. LWH: 75"x28 1/4"x46". Running surface: 60"x18". Required floor space: 75"x28 1/4". Weight: 165 lbs. Price: $2,800.00

Precor 720 Incline Exerciser ▶ Designed for full-body aerobic and anaerobic workouts, the 720 uses body weight as resistance, with 20 pin-lock settings for height adjustment. The steeper the incline setting, the more resistance. Made with the same attention to design and materials as other Precor products. Price: $500.00

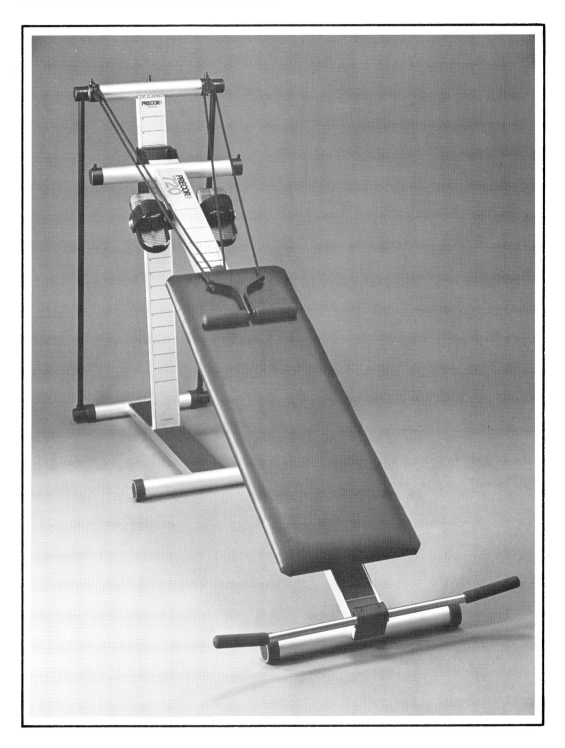

PSI-NordicTrack Co.

124 Columbia Court
Chaska, Minnesota 55318
1-800-328-5888, (612) 448-6987

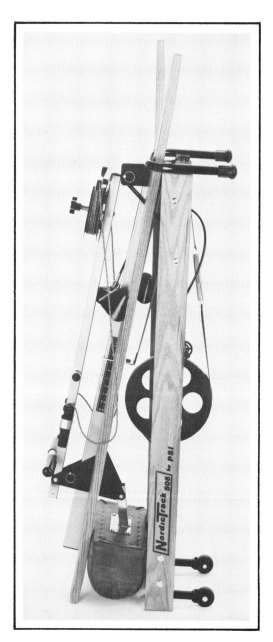

PSI-NordicTrack is the original maker of cross-country ski simulators. Its product-the NordicTrack-has caught on for home use as one of the most effective aerobic conditioning trainers available. Designed in 1975 by company founder Ed Pauls, a mechanical engineer and avid cross-country skier, the product has received rave reviews from exercise physiologists, athletic clubs, trainers and home users. PSI-NordicTrack only sells direct to the consumer, and offers a no-risk, 30-day trial. If the unit is returned, the company refunds purchase price and initial shipping and handling charges. Call or write for free brochures.

Cross-country skiers

NordicTrack This machine closely simulates the action of cross-country skiing. To operate the unit, a user pushes backward with the legs on two short skis that are supported by rollers located in tracks in the frame. As the skis move back and forth, the rollers drive a flywheel, which provides smooth, continuous action, even as weight is transferred from one foot to the other. Patented one-way clutches connect each ski's drive wheel to the flywheel, which provides correctly proportioned resistance for each leg (more resistance to the rear than forward). An adjustable belt tension strap allows an infinitely adjustable range of resistance for the skis. Toe pieces keep feet positioned on skis.

While the legs are working, the user works the upper body with a cord-type exerciser that simulates the arc-like motion of using ski poles. The cord drum has a disc brake that allows a wide range of tension adjustments. A hip level pad prevents the user from moving forward while exercising. The NordicTrack comes with speedometer/odometer. It folds and stands on end in a closet. LWH: (folded) 17"x15"x45". In operation, unit requires 2'x7'. Weight: 58 lbs. No assembly required. Price: $470.00. Shipping: $17.00. Accessories: Ski Pole Grips and Straps, $12.00; XR 210 Pulse Meter, $108.00

NordicTrack Pro The heavy-duty version of the NordicTrack has a heavier frame, deeper side boards, more damage resistant pad, wider front leg stance, and a numbered resistance setting for the arms. Requires 2'x7' operating area. LWH: (folded storage) 17"x23"x45". Price: $559.00. Shipping: $17.00.

◀ NordicTrack ▶

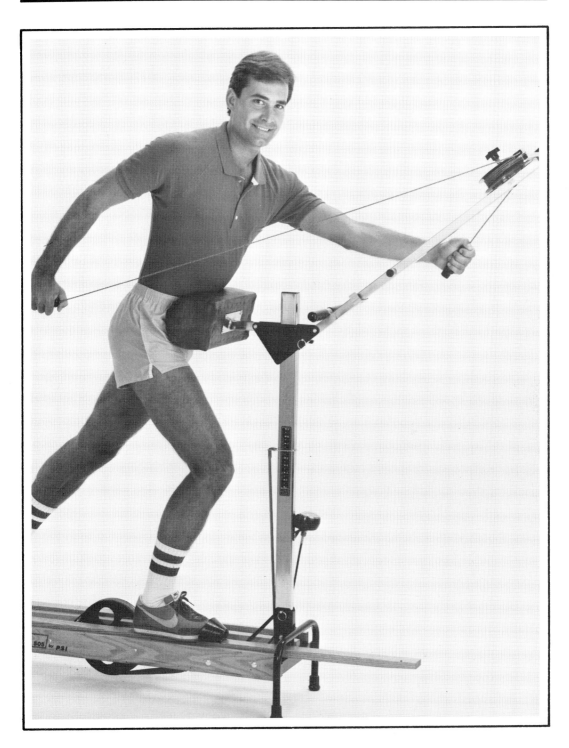

Soloflex
Hawthorn Farm Industrial Park
Hillsboro, Oregon 97124
1-800-547-8802
In Oregon, call collect, 640-8891

Soloflex is available direct from the manufacturer only. Endorsed by actor/body builder Arnold Schwarzenegger, it is attacting a large following. Soloflex users say it proves beyond a doubt that less is more when it comes to home gyms. Despite Soloflex's spare design, Mr. Schwarzenegger says it not only provides an "incredible" number of stations, but provides for exercises to be performed correctly in form and balance. Judge for yourself. The company offers a free (VHS) video brochure in addition to printed materials. If its provocative advertisements of well-muscled bodies don't make you sweat, the Soloflex itself certainly will.

Home gyms

Soloflex This is one machine that successfully blends beautiful design with unique function. Simple and elegant in matte-black and stainless steel, Soloflex almost qualifies as home sculpture. It has few moving parts and no weights. Instead, it relies on rubber weight straps for resistance. Each machine comes with 380 pounds of resistance in four weight strap sizes: five, ten, twenty-five and fifty pounders. The straps serve three functions: to provide resistance; to absorb shock between you and the machine; and to eliminate the danger of falling weight plates.

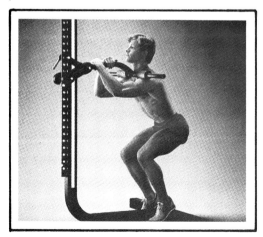

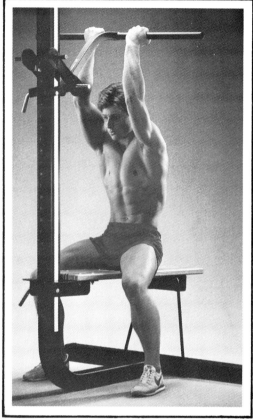

Soloflex

Soloflex is a simple machine with a movable, sparely padded incline bench and a curved bar. In its many configurations, the machine allows several types of sit-ups, bench press, leg press and military press, bicep curl, tricep pushdowns and extensions, chin-ups, pull-ups, squats, dips, and many other exercises. The machine provides for four different leg exercises.

Soloflex is constructed of steel, stainless steel and hardwood. One bolt secures the two sections of the mainframe. Weight straps and all parts are warranted for a full ten years. LWH: 4′ X 4′ X 6′. Weight: 170 lbs. The unit is shipped by motor freight with a $60.00 charge for shipping and handling. Shipping container dimensions: 6′ X 3′ X 7′′. Price: $565.00.

The company accepts major credit cards, money orders, and personal checks. Also available, subject to credit approval, is a time payment and a delayed credit card billing plan: $165.00 down and $50.00 per month for ten months.

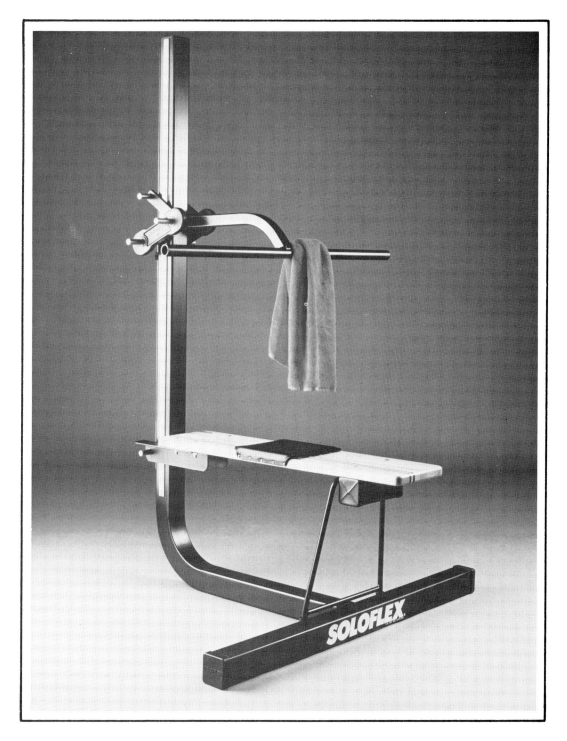

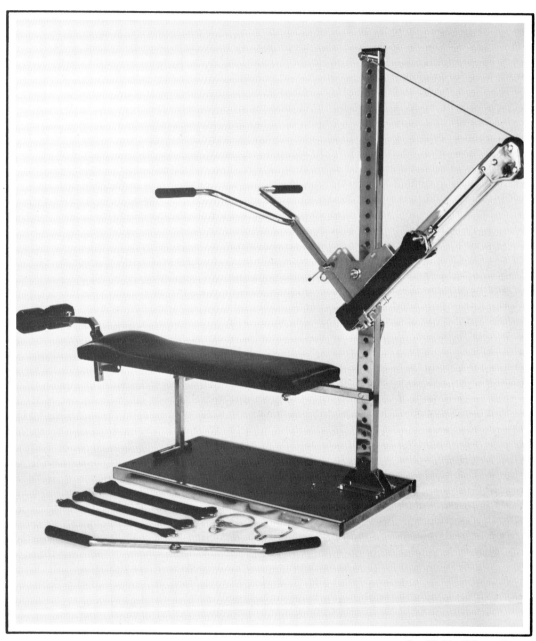

SupaFit Total Fitness System

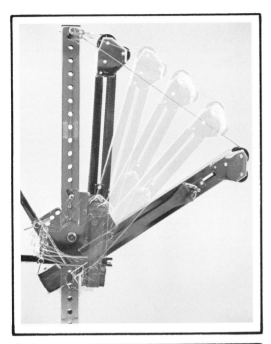

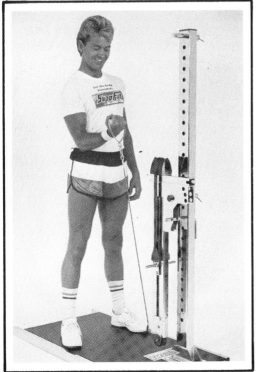

SupaFit Total Fitness Systems, Inc.
2615 W. Woodland Drive
Anaheim, California 92801
1-800-824-4319, (714) 952-3936

Designed in Australia by Andrew Dofel, engineer and ex-champion hammer thrower, the SupaFit Total Fitness System is one home gym that promises strong sales in the United States. It eliminates bulky weights and hydraulic resistance devices in favor of interchangeable resistance bands. A lightweight and functional design make it ideal for the home or office. Call or write for brochures and the name of the nearest dealer.

Home gyms

SupaFit Total Fitness System This machine is among the latest innovations in home gyms, incorporating elastic resistance bands that work with a lever assembly to provide resistance up to 480 lbs. The SupaFit system is free-standing, weighing about 130 lbs., and is capable of more than 40 exercises to trim, tone and condition the entire body. Made of heavy-duty, chrome plated steel, the system incorporates seven components: a base platform; column; fulcrum assembly; lifting bar; lat bar; padded bench; and a leg extension attachment. The system comes with four tension bands that are fully socketed and can be secured at desired tension levels with locking knobs. The product requires an exercise area of about 3 1/2' by 5'. Height is about 6', and width (at base) is 24''. Price: $695.00

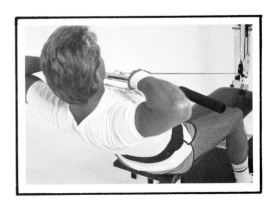

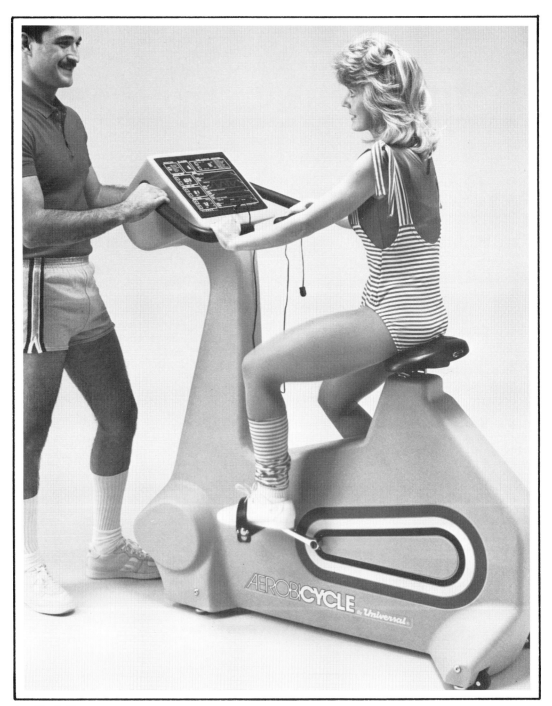

Aerobicycle II

Universal is one of the most respected and oldest names in physical conditioning equipment. The company also is in the forefront of the home fitness market. Not only does it manufacture an extensive line of fitness products, it distributes several other manufacturers' lines, such as the Monark line of exercise cycles, Avita products, and the Concept II rower. (Avita and Concept II products are listed elswhere in *HomeWork-out.*) Universal products also are widely available through all types of retail outlets. Call or write for free brochures.

Exercise cycles

Aerobicycle I   This advanced aerobic conditioning system is designed with three, pre-programmed exercise modes that also monitor your exercise progress. Just start pedaling, and depress the exercise mode of your choice: steady climb, rolling hills, or constant rpm. The machine takes you through a course of exercise, telling you the time remaining in your exercise session, how many calories you are burning, your pulse rate (taken from an earlobe clip sensor), the cycle's work load level, and the pedal speed. The system runs on pedal power, and requires no external electrical power source. All working parts, except the pedals, are fully enclosed. The unit comes with two-position handlebars, adjustable seat, case-hardened crank, and maintenance free construction. Price: $2,160.00

Aerobicycle II   This model is exactly like the Aerobicycle I, except it has two additional pre-programmed exercise modes on its console: pulse rate training, and fitness test. The pulse training mode automatically adjusts the cycle's work load to maintain the target pulse rate that you establish. The fitness test mode furnishes the user with his or her aerobic fitness level in percentile ranking (based on YMCA national norms). Price: $2,480.00

Monark Home Ergometer (865)   This ergometer cycle is ideal for individual training and fitness testing. A console instrument panel shows brake resistance (in watts), in addition to speedometer/odometer, and timer. The frame is made of heavy gauge tube steel. The cycle features a heavy flywheel that is braked with a tension-adjustable nylon resistance strap. The cycle collapses for easy storage. LWH: (with handlebar at maximum height) 38"x15 3/4"x49". Saddle height range: 29 1/2" to 42". Color: white. Price: $460.00

Universal Fitness Equipment
50 Commercial Street
Plainview, Long Island, NY 11803
1-800-645-7554, (516) 349-8600

Monark Home Ergometer 865

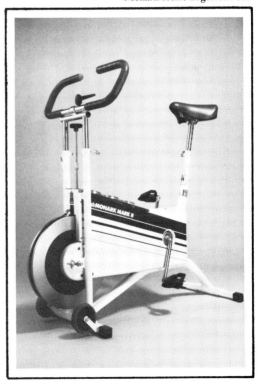

Monark Trim Guide 2000
A multi-function heart monitor with choice of earlobe sensor or highly accurate electrocardiogram (ECG) chest belt. Features pre-set memory function for high/low heart rate and watt settings, with audible alarm when user strays from target zone. Monitor displays calorie consumption and calorie consumption rate, elapsed time, work load (in watts), and weak battery. Mounting bracket allows monitor to be used with all exercise equipment. Price: $199.00; optional ECG belt, $25.00

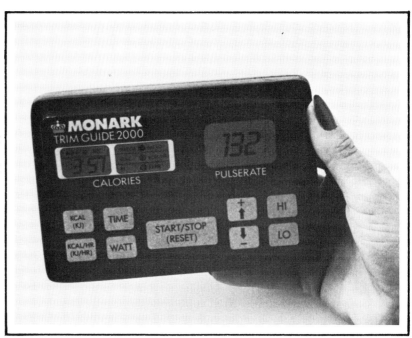

Monark Pro II 867

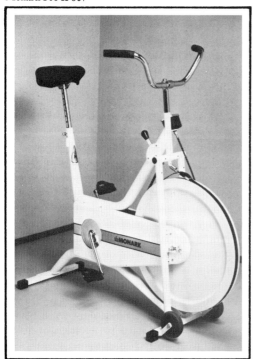

Monark Pro II (867) This model is built to withstand the demands of heavy use. Heavy gauge frame construction and extra large, well balanced flywheel ensure durability and smooth pedaling action. The cycle features adjustable nylon tension strap with seven resistance settings, and adjustable seat and handlebars. LWH: (with handlebar at maximum height) 44"x23"x42 1/2". Color: white. Price: $495.00

Home gyms

Power-Pak 300 This versatile, free-standing gym offers six standard exercise stations, and is capable of more than 100 exercises. Stations include chest/shoulder press; high pulley; low pulley; thigh/knee exerciser; abdominal conditioner; leg squat attachment ($140.00); and leg press attachment ($76.00).

The Power-Pak 300 comes with a choice of 100, 180 or 260 lb. captured weight stacks in black or chrome finish. Extra weights can be added to the 100 and 180 lb. stacks. The pulley and thigh/knee stations share the same weight stack as the chest/shoulder press, and are attached to the lifting mechanism by a quick-release lever. Because of the double pulley design, however, the maximum weight resistance for these stations is half that of the chest/shoulder press. The Power-Pak 300 is made of 2"

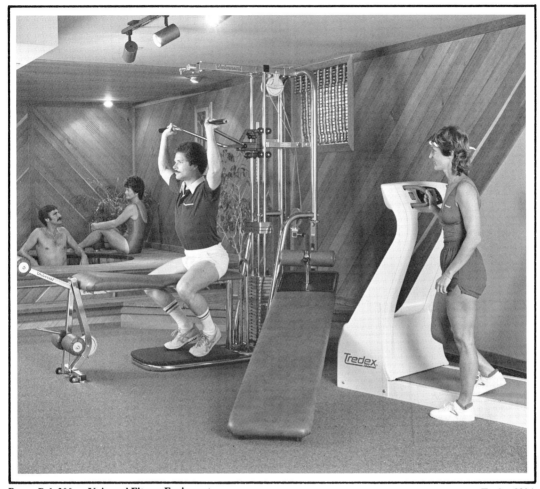

Power-Pak 300 —Universal Fitness Equipment

Tredex 2924

Treadmills

round, nickel-chrome plated steel, and outfitted with well padded Naugahyde upholstery. The unit also features high-test steel cables, and self-aligning nylon alloy bushings on the lifting assembly. The Power-Pak fits into a compact area. LWH: 96″x96″x84″. Price: (basic unit with 180 lb. black weight stack) $1,735.00; thigh/knee unit, $595.00; flat bench, $150.00. Price includes delivery.

Power-Pak 250 This is a wall-mounted version of the Power-Pak 300. It requires slightly less floor space. LWH: 82″x96″x84″. Price: (basic unit with 180 lb. black weight stack) $1,032.00; thigh/knee unit, $595.00; flat bench, $150.00. Price includes delivery.

Tredex 2924 This state-of-the-art, motorized treadmill features a computerized control panel that shows speed, running time, distance and pace per mile in an easy-to-read digital display. A direct drive (DC) motor provides infinite speed control up to eight mph, and runs on standard household current. Special safety handles provide hand holds when starting and stopping. They also serve as emergency shut-off when pushed downward. A special non-strech belt travels across a flat surface for comfortable running. A sleek, low profile makes mounting and dismounting easy. LWH: 81″x25″x50″. Weight: 230 lbs. Price: $2,995.00

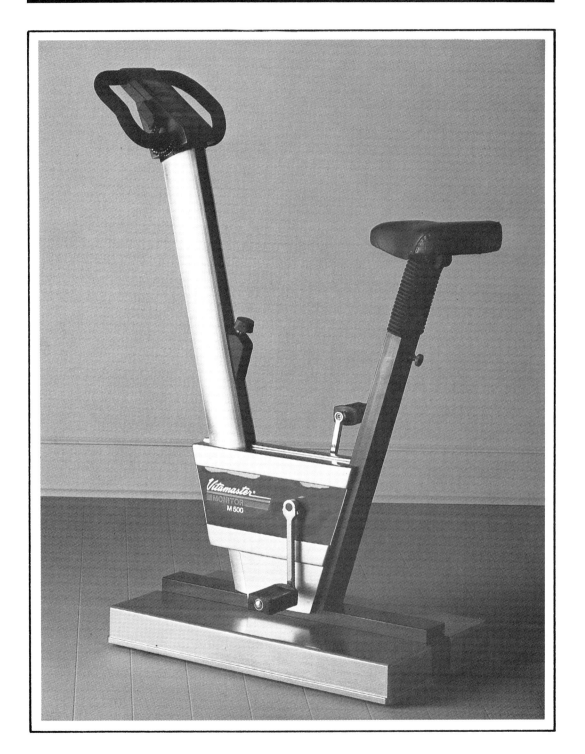

Vitamaster

Division of Allegheny International Exercise
Co.
Hwy. 321, Bypass North
Lincolnton, North Carolina 28092
1-800-848-2348, (704) 735-6582

Vitamaster is the largest manufacturer of exercise cycles and a pioneering manufacturer of home exercise equipment. Known for innovation, craftsmanship, and quality, the company has taken a leadership position in developing "total fitness" home systems. Call the company for brochures about products and for dealers nearest you.

Exercise cycles

500M, 400M, 300M Monitor Exercise Cycles

These top-of-the-line cycles have totally electronic consoles that provide a workout with a readout. Each has a twenty-five pound flywheel with adjustable web strap resistance system. Flywheels are vertically mounted on the 300M and horizontally mounted on 400M and 500M models. Each cycle has adjustable seats and handlebars, fully enclosed gear-box drives, padded seats, and foam handgrips. (The 300M is chain driven.)

The console on the 300M has LED display of time, speed, and distance. The 400M console has an additional display of pulse rate (taken from a finger clip sensor). The 500M console has an additional display of pulse rate, calories expended, and calories per hour (work load). Each console offers selection of display mode in eight-second intervals or continuous readout. Displays automatically shut down after five minutes to conserve batteries.

The cycles have sturdy 3" X ½" rectangular steel tube frames, and maintenance-free gear box and flywheel operation. LWH: (maximum) 30" X 15" X 47". Weight: 65 to 75 lbs. Colors: Silver, black with bright graphics. Price: (300M) $350.00; (400M) $600.00; (500M) $850.00

◀ **Monitor 500M**

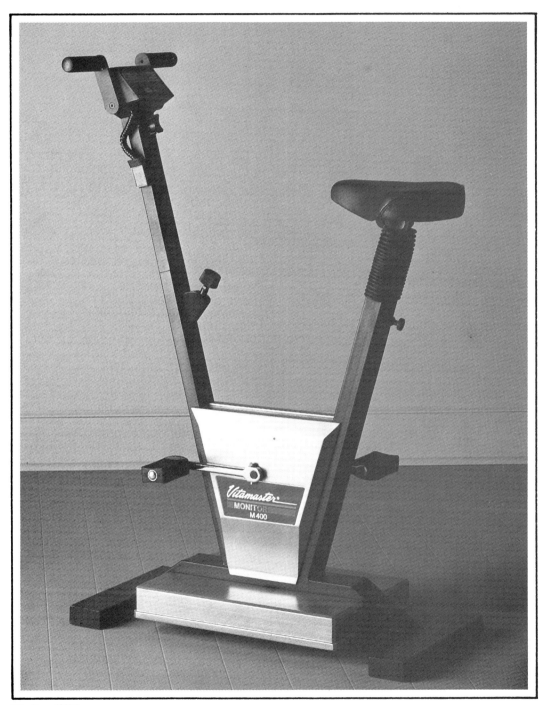

Monitor 400M

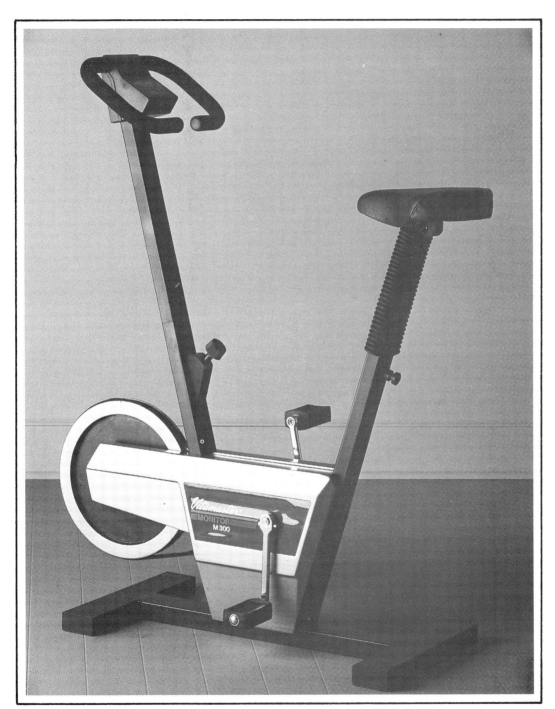

Monitor 300M —Vitamaster

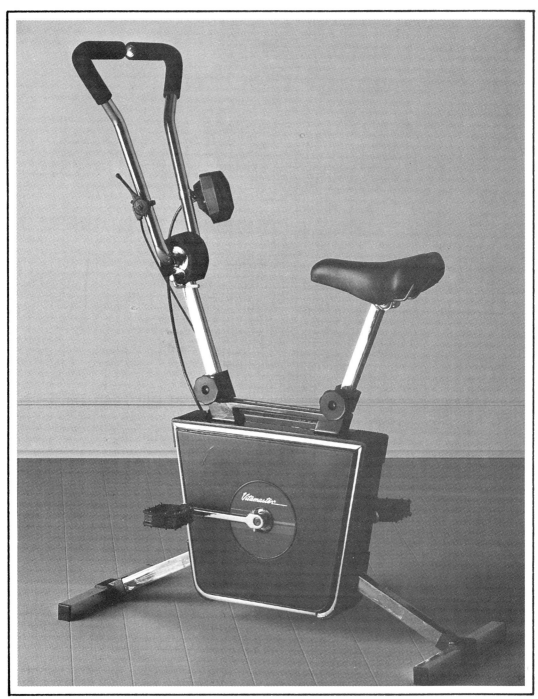

Hide-A-Cycle 820H

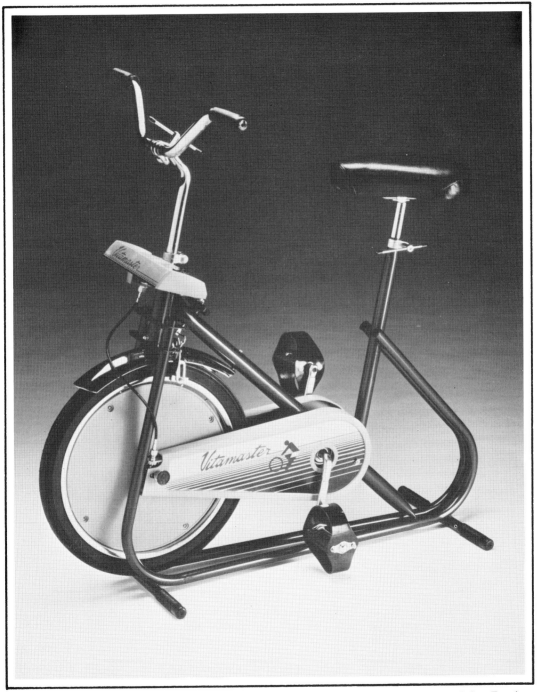

Deluxe Exercisers

Pro*1000 Monitor This exercise cycle also has a fully electronic console that measures performance in time, speed, distance, calories per hour (work load), calories expended, and pulse rate. Data appear at eight-second intervals on LED displays. The cycle is built of 1¼'' tube steel frame with extra wide front/rear legs. It includes a thirty-nine-pound steel flywheel with precision bearings and adjustable tension control. Colors: silver, chrome. Price: $705.00

Exercisers For the budget-conscious, several models are available in standard and custom designs. Well-constructed but nothing fancy, these cycles offer a variety of consoles, speedometer/odometers, and timers (including four-function electronic console). Price range: $155.00 to $340.00

Dual Action Trainer If you like rowing and pedaling, this is the cycle for you. Handlebars lock in two positions for pedaling only. They unlock for use with the shock absorber tension device that allows rowing motion. Both actions may be performed separately or together. The frame is 1½'' welded fourteen-gauge tube steel with protective floor guards. A combination speedometer/odometer and thirty-minute timer are featured. Color: desert beige. Weight: 51 lbs. Price: $275.00

Home gyms

Station One Station One is an exerciser with many strong points. Designed to exercise all muscle groups, the gym is capable of more than fifty exercises. Station One may be wall-mounted or free-standing with optional accessory. The system comes with a 110-pound weight stack (in ten-pound increments) that glides up and down on steel rail. Extra weight sets are available. Features include an adjustable inclined padded bench; eight-position handlebar; height adjustable undercarriage; padded headboard; three-inch upholstered arm/leg developer, and more. Accessories include double-handled pulley rope, ankle and wrist pulley belt, and lat bar. A weight unit has wheels for easy movability. The entire unit folds to within fifteen inches of wall for compact storage. Price: (basic unit) $485.00; (free-standing unit) $210.00; (50 lb. accessory weights) $75.00

Station One —Vitamaster

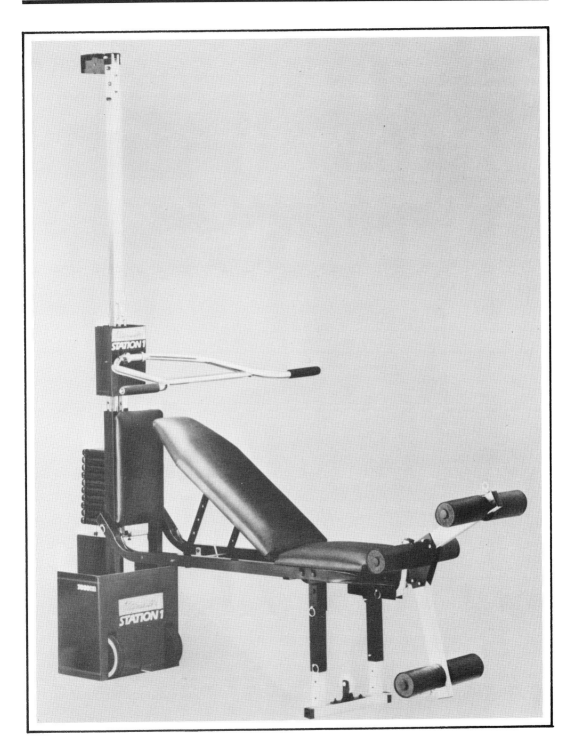

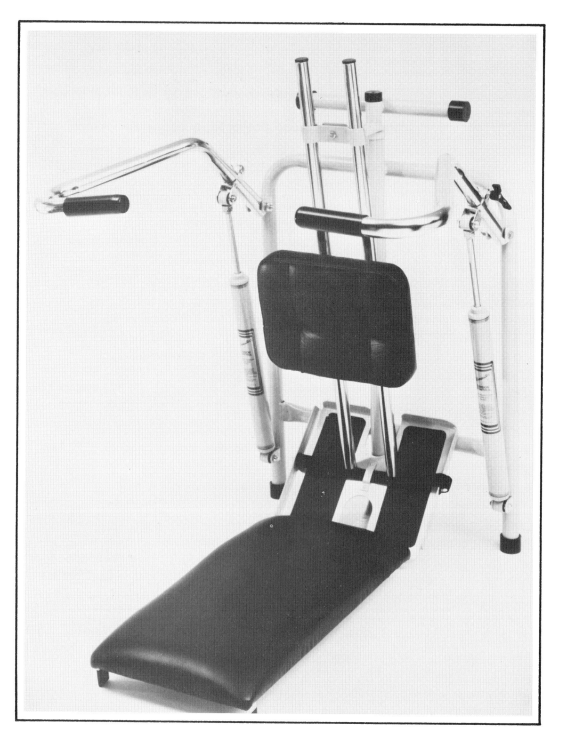

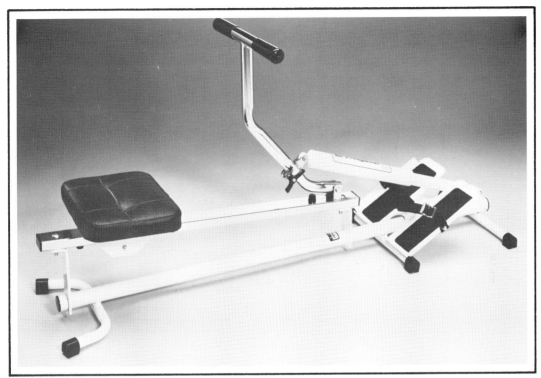

Standard Hydraulic Rower (RM-4)

MA*500 This is a "Multi-Action Gym" that can be used in a horizontal position as rowing machine, or with addition of backrest for vertical multi-action exercises. Hydraulic cylinders allow independent action of each arm with three tension adjustments. The telescoping frame (made of 1½" tube steel) adjusts to any person's height. The padded seat is mounted on nylon rollers and the molded footrest has adjustable nylon straps. The unit folds up for flat storage. Colors: desert beige with graphics, and chrome, black vinyl seat/backrest. Weight: 43.5 lbs. Price: $185.00

Rowers

Standard Hydraulic Rower (RM-4) This rower has only one, center-mounted hydraulic tension device. It folds and stands for compact storage. No assembly required. Weight: 34 lbs. Color: white with bright graphics. Price: $145.00

MA*500 —Vitamaster

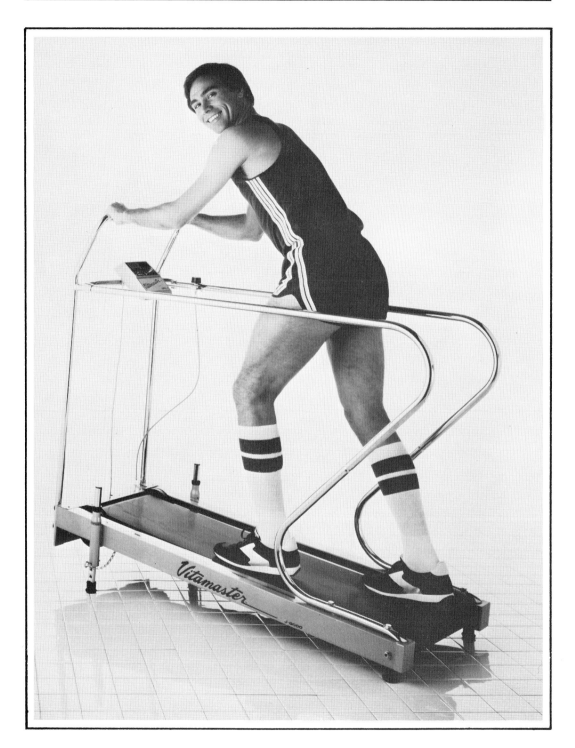

◀ Pro＊6000

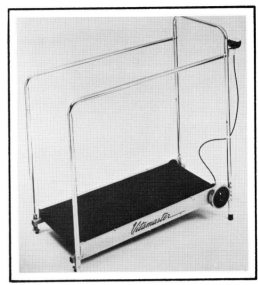

Treadmaster Joggers

Treadmills

750M Monitor Jogger   This motorized jogger features a flat-bed running surface powered by a 1.5 hp motor. Running speeds from zero to eight mph are controlled by a console switch. Unit also has a pull-on/push-off emergency switch. An electronic console gives LED readings for time, speed, and distance. The unit is constructed of a sturdy anodized aluminum frame. Weight: 500 lbs. Color: silver, black with bright graphics. Price: Approx. $1,800.00

Pro＊6000   This top-of-the-line manual treadmill has all the extras. It features added length for full stride; infinite tension adjustment control; adjustable tread surface angle that imitates level, uphill, or steep incline; flat running surface (no rollers); heavy-duty front and rear flywheel drums for smooth action; and chrome front and full-length side rails. Pro＊6000 comes with speedometer/reset odometer and timer. Weight: 120 lbs. Price: $575.00

Treadmaster Joggers   Four manual models are available with a variety of features and prices. These models have continuous vinyl mats and drum drives with dual four-pound flywheels. Deluxe model has a curved bed design with graduated incline. All treadmaster models are also available with flat bed surface. All offer adjustable inclines for level, uphill, and steep settings. Various speedometer/odometer consoles and timers are available. Price range: (custom models) $275.00 to $310.00; (deluxe model) $415.00

The West Bend Company

400 Washington St., P.O. Box 278
West Bend, Wisconsin 53095
(414) 334-2311

A newcomer to the home fitness scene, West Bend has become a major player by acquiring a few innovative smaller manufacturers. The company has used its superior marketing and distribution skills to bring several promising and unique products into wider distribution.

Home gyms

Total Gym   Two models (the Pro and Pro-Plus) are available with slight variations to accommodate anyone from the beginner to the serious athlete. Both are free-standing and are constructed of heavy-gauge steel tubing with chrome plating and black epoxy finish.

Each model is capable of more than seventy exercises designed to promote strength, aerobic conditioning, and flexibility. The system can be used to train for active sports or for bodybuilding. The resistance principle uses the body's own weight as the workload. You exercise by sliding up and down on a padded glide board. Workload may be increased or decreased by adjusting the height of the board. Both models also feature a weight-lifting frame to increase resistance load. Another feature is compact storage; when not in use, the units fold up. Descriptions of both models follow.

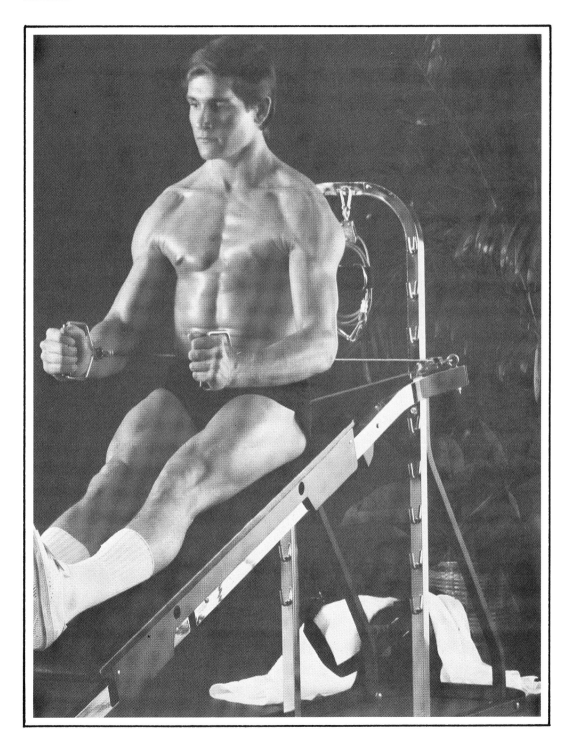

Pro Nine glideboard levels plus a built-in weight bar gives user the option of almost unlimited resistance. (Higher levels provide more resistance.) Other features include two-handle arm pulley, padded glide board, swivel foot holder, and standard leg cuff for lower body exercises. The unit folds into a forty-eight-inch (deep) floor space when not in use. Price: $495.00

Pro Plus The deluxe Total Gym with all features and extra heavy-duty construction, Pro Plus features eleven resistance levels, padded glideboard, padded swivel foot holder, deluxe leg cuff, chrome squat stand, and weight lifting frame. The unit folds into a forty-eight-inch (deep) floor space for storage. Price $499.00

Accessories You can upgrade, replace and / or add features to either Total Gym model. Accessories include:

Deluxe Leg Cuff Leather band, lamb's wool lining, and Velcro strap. Includes cable and pulley. $39.95

Standard Leg Cuff Wide Velcro strap with soft inner lining. Includes cable and pulley. $25.95

Squat Stand Hooks to the base of the Total Gym. Includes chrome plated steel tubing and padded foot board. $44.95

Curl Bench Padded bench slides on top of glideboard to support arms while exercising. $59.95

Weight Lifting Bar Includes thirty-four-inch bar (no weights) that slips through frame. $12.95

Swivel Foot Holder Heavily padded holder is located at top of glide rails. Velcro straps hold feet securely during exercise. $28.95

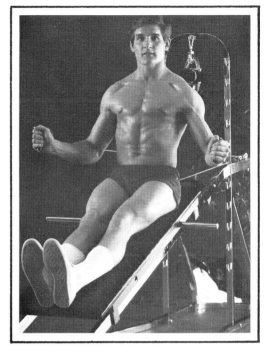

5100XL Rowing Machine ▼

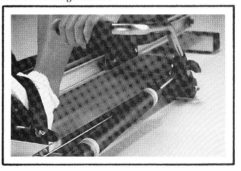

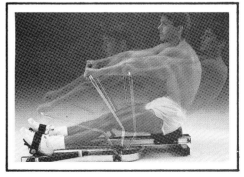

Rowers

5100XL Rowing Machine This unit combines precision engineering with quality construction. It features a cushioned, anatomically designed seat with smooth rolling action; single-beam, anodized aluminum rail with internal track; and pivoting foot pedals with self-adhering, adjustable bands. Chrome-plated steel rowing arms feature fingertip tension adjustments. Dual hydraulic cylinders ensure smooth, constant resistance. Great for rowing, this machine also is capable of many upper body exercises. Price: $249.00

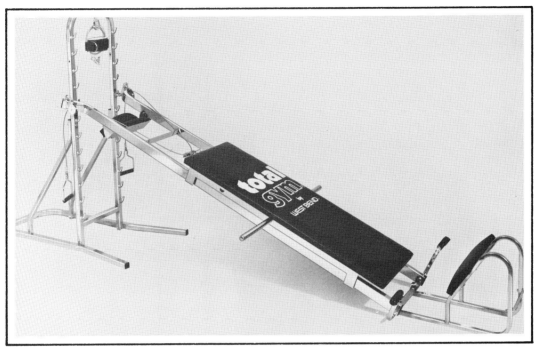

▼ Pro-Plus ▲   ▼ Pro —The West Bend Co.

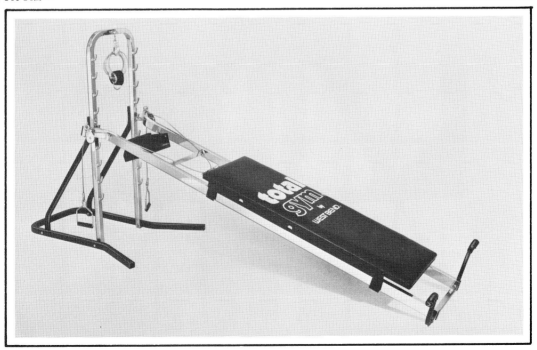

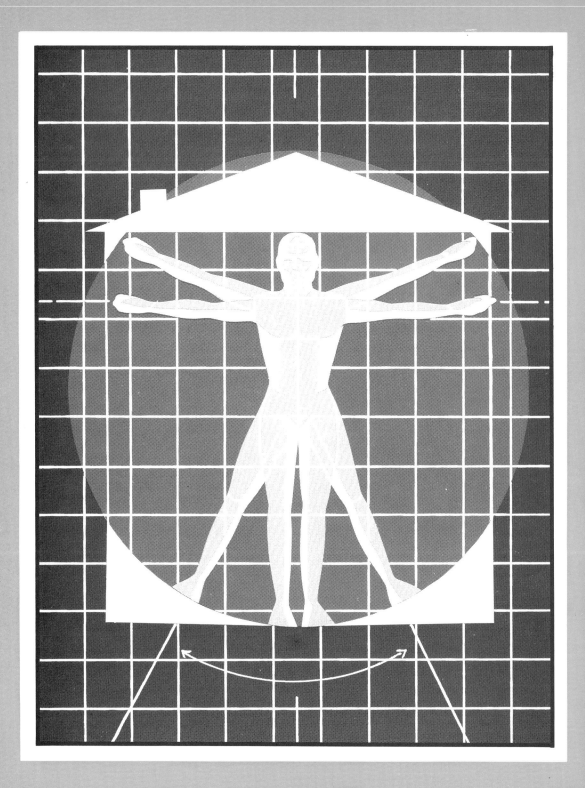

Exercise

Muscles, muscles, muscles

The basic function of your muscles is really very simple—to contract. Your every movement—from the blink of an eye to a sprinting run—can be reduced to this simple process.

Your muscles are arranged so that each muscle, or muscle group, has a counterpart muscle, or group that pulls in a different direction. When you move an extremity one way, an opposing set of muscles allows you to pull it back. These opposing sets of muscles work together to give your body a full range of motion.

For example, when you slowly raise your lower arm from a hanging position, palm up and bent at the elbow, the bicep muscle at the front of your upper arm contracts. Try it. When you turn your hand over and slowly lower your arm, the tricep muscle at the back of your upper arm contracts. Its contraction opposes the contraction of the bicep.

Muscle types

For most people, the word *muscle* brings to mind prominent muscles of the arms, legs, and trunk. These are skeletal muscles. While they comprise most of the body's muscle mass, there is quite a bit more.

Your body actually has three types of muscle. *Smooth muscles* line the insides of your intestines and are found throughout the circulatory system. You have very little direct control over these muscles. Consequently, there is not much you can do directly to improve them through home fitness.

The *heart* is a muscle, similar to skeletal muscles, except that its fibers are woven together in an interlacing network rather than running alongside each other. It also is similar to smooth muscles in that an adequate stimulus is passed from fiber to fiber.

The heart is unique because it has special cells (called ''pacemakers'') that generate a tiny electrical current. These cells set off a wavelike contraction that passes through the entire muscle, pumping blood throughout the body.

Unlike skeletal muscles, the heart contracts automatically. You have little direct control over its function, unless you are a master of yoga. But you do have considerable indirect control over your heart. You can improve its endurance and strength through exercises requiring a high level of repetition. Treadmills, exercise cycles, rowers, rebounders, and other pieces of home fitness equipment, are designed to condition and improve the function of the heart and lungs.

Skeletal muscles

Skeletal muscles, the third type of muscle in your body, are under your voluntary control. It is these muscles that many pieces of home fitness equipment are designed to tone and strengthen.

Skeletal muscles are composed of long, cylindrical fibers, each of which is wrapped in a connective sheath. Although they are all bundled together in a tough casing, each fiber acts independently of its neighbors.

When you regularly exercise using increasing levels of resistance, several things happen. The muscle fibers begin to expand and thicken, and blood supply and nerve stimulation to individual fibers and to the local muscle area improve. Eventually, your body is able to call more fibers into each muscular contraction, thereby increasing your strength.

The results you get from exercise depend, to a large extent, on the types of muscle fibers involved. There are at least three different types of fibers in the skeletal muscles: red fibers, white fibers, and an intermediate category that you could think of as ''pink'' fibers.

White muscle fiber is capable of

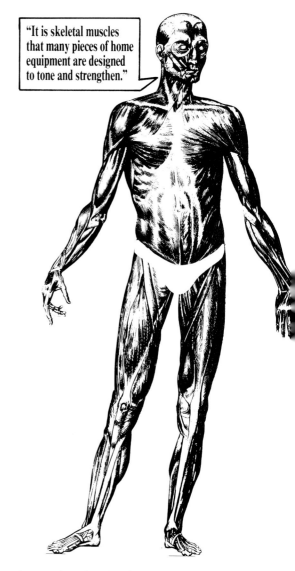

"It is skeletal muscles that many pieces of home equipment are designed to tone and strengthen."

tremendous bursts of strength, after which it tires easily. Red muscle fiber, on the other hand, has great endurance but is capable of producing much less overall strength. ''Pink'' fiber is capable of being conditioned through different types of exercise to resemble and act something like either red or white fibers.

To help you understand the capabilities of each fiber type, a useful comparison is to think of the chicken. A chicken's leg muscles are composed almost entirely of red muscle fiber (dark meat) and its wings and breast of white muscle fiber (white meat). These muscle types are ideal adaptations for the chicken's method of survival. When in danger, the chicken needs explosive strength (white fibers) to fly, and yet it cannot fly very far because white fibers have little endurance. The chicken, as a ground bird, relies on its feet and the great endurance of its legs (red fibers) to carry it to safety.

Unlike chickens, people have a mixture of fiber types—red, pink, and white—in each muscle. Each of us is born with a genetically determined ratio of these different muscle fibers that no amount of exercise will change. In other words, if your muscles have a high concentration of white fibers, you have the innate capacity to build great strength and muscle size. Most bodybuilders fit this description. If your muscles tend to have a high concentration of red fibers, you have the capability of excelling in exercise that requires endurance. Marathon runners and cross-country skiers generally have this quality. Most people, however, are genetically in between, with neither muscle fiber type being dominant.

Regardless of muscle fiber composition, regular home exercise can help to improve your muscular strength and endurance. In other words, with suitable training, white fibers become more enduring and red fibers become stronger. And "pink" fibers go along with the rest.

Basic training

There are many different training methods for improving your physical condition. The intent of some is to build muscles. For others, the goal is to increase muscular strength and power, or to improve endurance, motor coordination, flexibility, and speed.

Likewise, most home exercise machines are designed with specific purposes in mind. They are built to help you improve your physical performance in a number of predictable ways, if you give them a healthy investment of your time and sweat.

> **phys·ical fit·ness,** adaptations that are conducive to long term good health.
>
> ❧

Don't fool yourself into thinking that all machines work alike or produce the same results. They don't. Some are designed to tone you up all over; some are meant to work only on muscles in specific areas. Others are engineered to improve the condition of your heart and lungs.

This chapter will help you to discover what regular exercise on home fitness machines can do for you. It examines the individual components of physical fitness as they relate to various home exercise machines.

First, some definitions are in order, starting with the term *physical fitness*. According to the dictionary, *fitness* means "adapted to a purpose." While that's a good partial definition of *physical fitness*, it still comes up short for our purposes. It fails to specify for *what* the fitness is adapted.

For example, you may be well adapted to sitting behind the wheel of a car as your primary mode of transportation, or to spending hours each day behind a desk or in front of a television. And yet, these types of adaptations would not help you become physically fit.

A better definition of physical fitness is "adaptations that are conducive to long-term good health." Such adaptations might include improved heart and lung capacity, improved muscular strength and endurance, greater balance and coordination, and a few others.

But this definition still would not be complete without some mention of time. Your body's adaptations take place over weeks, months, and years. In this respect, physical fitness is an on-going process during which your body continually adapts to greater or lesser amounts of exercise.

The elements of fitness

Now that you have a working definition of fitness, it's time to look at its individual qualities:

- *Muscular strength*
- *Muscular endurance*
- *Aerobic endurance*
- *Anaerobic endurance*
- *Speed*
- *Flexibility*
- *Motor coordination*

Each of these elements is a factor in your home fitness program. But don't make the mistake of thinking that each element is distinct from the others. In truth, all of the elements are so closely interwoven they are nearly impossible to separate. This section breaks apart some aspects of physical fitness just to give you a picture of how the elements work together.

Muscular strength

Muscular strength comes from only one source, work. Your muscles grow in girth when they are trained with resistance exercise. Home weight machines, free weights, and other devices that permit gradual increases in resistance are excellent means of improving muscular strength.

Your muscle fibers gradually adapt to the increased weight (or resistance) by expanding and thickening. Muscle growth as a result of progressive resistance training is called *hypertrophy.*

Muscular shrinkage, or *atrophy,* is the reverse effect, and it is caused by disuse. Atrophy begins when you stop forcing your muscles to do work. If you have ever looked at someone's arm or leg after recovery from a broken bone and their cast has been removed, you have seen the effects of atrophy. Muscles shrivel, losing most of their tone and strength. While it may not be as obvious, atrophy begins taking its toll on your

muscles if you work for long hours behind a desk or if you simply stop using them through inactivity.

Just how much strength you possess in a particular muscle depends on three things: the number of muscle fibers it is composed of; how many fibers are involved in a muscle contraction; and the thickness and capacity of each fiber.

One measure of strength is the amount of *work* that your muscles can perform (measured as force times distance). For example, if you lift 100 pounds to a height of five feet, you have done 500 foot-pounds of work. Another measure of strength is *muscle power,* the ability to produce force at varying rates of speed. For example, if two men are each capable of lifting 300 pounds, but one lifts the weight twice as fast as the other, the faster one exerts twice as much muscle power. Power is usually described in terms of *horsepower.* One unit of horsepower equals the ability to produce 550 foot-pounds per second.

Muscular endurance

Muscular endurance is the ability to persist in a physical activity, such as lifting a weight. Improving muscular endurance is important in a home fitness program because it reduces the tendency of your muscles to tire easily (*muscle fatigue*) when you work or play. Probably the best way to improve muscle strength and endurance is through progressive resistance training with single- and multi-station home gyms.

Muscle endurance, in truth, is almost impossible to separate from general endurance involving your body's *overall* physical response to exercise. (General endurance is described in this section under *Aerobic endurance.*) To separate the two, many refer to muscular endurance as *local muscular endurance.* This simply limits discussion to *a muscle,* or a group of muscles.

Muscular endurance is limited partly by your

ability to take pain, and by your motivation to put more effort into your exercising. Unless your goal is to become a top athlete, however, there is no reason to push yourself to the point of actual pain in a home fitness program. You will know that your muscles are reaching the limits of their endurance when you begin to feel a slight burning sensation. This is the result of chemical changes that cause muscle fatigue.

The other factors that affect muscular endurance are strength, energy stored in the

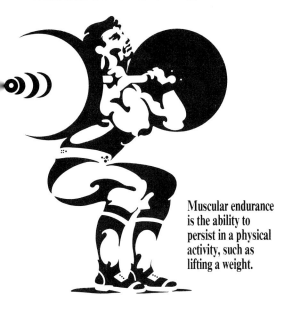

Muscular endurance is the ability to persist in a physical activity, such as lifting a weight.

muscle itself, and blood circulation. Put simply, when your muscles are working extra hard, they quickly use up energy supplies that are stored alongside individual muscle fibers. Because muscular contraction temporarily blocks incoming blood circulation, there is no replenishment of energy supplies and oxygen. Regular progressive resistance workouts improve the muscles' ability to use energy supplies, and increase their tolerance to chemical changes causing fatigue.

The relationship is close between muscular endurance, muscular strength, and power. Studies on athletic training have shown that improving muscular strength is the first priority

in improving muscular endurance. More strength allows muscles to perform the same level of work at lower levels of activity. Power training comes into play because it has been shown that high repetition exercises with light work loads are not as effective in improving muscular endurance as low repetition exercises with heavier work loads.

As a final note, there appears to be little difference in muscular endurance due to sex, when differences in strength are ruled out. Neither does age appear to be a major factor in muscular endurance, although it seems to be a factor in the rate of muscle fatigue. Temperature is a factor in muscle endurance and muscle fatigue. When the thermometer is up, your muscles have less endurance and tire more easily.

Aerobic endurance

Aerobic endurance is measured by your ability to do sustained work, such as running, cycling, and other forms of active exercise. Your body's ability to take in oxygen and transport it to the muscles, where it is used to process energy, is the most important physical aspect of aerobic endurance. But equally important is the endurance limit that is set mentally—your motivation and willingness to work hard.

Both the physical and mental aspects of aerobic endurance can be improved dramatically through regular workouts on a treadmill, exercise cycle, rower, rebounder, and other pieces of home fitness equipment. These forms of exercise require general endurance, because they place a work load on a combination of muscle groups, and on the action of your body's central systems— the heart, lungs and others. As the level of exercise intensity rises, there is an increase in the heart rate, the rate of breathing, blood pressure, sweating, and other processes. In other words, aerobic exercises get your whole body moving.

What actually happens during aerobic

exercise is highly complex. But it can be simplified into a process that begins with the body at rest, all body processes at normal levels. When aerobic exercise begins, there is a lag between the oxygen required by the muscles for metabolizing energy, and the ability of the heart, lungs, and circulatory system to provide it. While the body is adapting to the intensity of the exercise, the muscles are able to function for a very short time on energy sources that do not require oxygen. These are called anaerobic energy

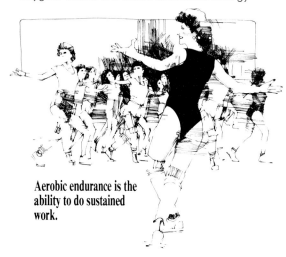

Aerobic endurance is the ability to do sustained work.

sources. The energy supplied by anaerobic sources starts high and levels off within minutes, however, and the aerobic machinery takes over as it heats up. When you finish exercising, the aerobic machinery continues functioning at a high level for several minutes until oxygen is restored to normal levels in the muscles.

You can see from this description of the body's response to aerobic exercise why it is so important to warm up before exercising and cool down afterwards. Because your body takes a few minutes to respond to exercise (assuming you don't overload it), and a few minutes to get back to resting levels when you finish, it is a good idea to work with—not against—these physical processes in your exercise routine.

How quickly your body responds to an

aerobic activity—climbing a set of stairs, for example—depends on the capacity of your lungs, the strength and output of your heart, the dynamics of your circulatory system, and the oxygen-carrying capacity of your blood. These factors set the limits on the amount of oxygen your body is able to use during aerobic exercise. To some degree, many of these limits are genetically determined. That is why not just anybody is capable of becoming a world-class athlete.

But regular use of home fitness equipment—treadmills, rowers, stationary cycles—can bring about *substantial* increases in your aerobic capacity. This can improve nearly every aspect of your life, giving you more energy and quicker recovery from daily exertions.

Regular aerobic exercise can give you a lower resting heart rate, improved breathing and heart function, faster response to and recovery from exercise, and improved general endurance, among other benefits. All you need is the motivation to work hard during about three sessions per week.

Anaerobic endurance

Anaerobic energy sources provide the muscles with fast fuel for explosive bursts of energy. Unlike aerobic endurance, which comes into play during sustained activity, *anaerobic endurance* is important in the ability to create high levels of work (force over a distance) in a short period of time.

Anaerobic endurance could be thought of as the ability to quickly move your body weight over a short distance, as in a sprint run. This is important in most active sports, such as football, handball, baseball, and basketball, where repeated jumping, sprinting, and overall quickness are vital to winning. Anaerobic endurance is particularly important to weightlifters, who may depend entirely on anaerobic energy reserves when lifting a huge weight.

It is important to note that the fast fuel of anaerobic energy cannot be separated from the slower chemical break-down of aerobic fuel. Your body uses both processes in a kind of loop to extract the most energy out of digested foods—carbohydrates, sugars, and fats. The end product of this chemical process (at the cellular level) are carbon dioxide and water, which are carried away by the bloodstream.

As noted in the section on aerobic endurance, your body relies on *anaerobic* energy sources when you *start* a workout, but these sources are depleted within minutes, after which your body needs rest (and oxygen) to replenish anaerobic reserves. You can, however, condition your body to a higher level of anaerobic endurance by working out regularly with weights, or with a variety of the home gyms shown in *HomeWork-out*. This is called strength, or *power*, training, and it involves high-speed, intensive workouts for short periods, alternated with periods of rest.

Power training has several effects: it causes muscle growth, it improves the supply of the fast fuel needed for anaerobic energy, and it improves the muscles' ability to use available energy sources. Studies also have shown that continuous *aerobic* training has a positive effect on an individual's *anaerobic* capacity.

Speed

Speed is defined as *the rate of motion,* but there is a lot more that can be said about this important quality. Speed, in the physical sense, is what you get when you apply force to a mass. The resulting velocity is determined by how much force acts on how much mass, minus resistance from negative forces, such as gravity, friction, and air resistance.

Using the human body as the *mass,* and muscle power as the *force* in this equation, an increase in speed could be gained either from increasing the muscle *force,* or from decreasing resistance. Assuming resistance and other factors remain constant, it is only logical that improving muscle force (strength) is the answer to improving an individual's speed.

Just exactly how an individual could best go about improving speed is a matter of some controversy. Gains in speed have been demonstrated to result purely from strength training, such as working out on home gyms, and from training that duplicates the type of movement being tested. Examples of the latter case might include improved strength from stationary cycling or from a rowing machine, and resulting improvements in speed during cycle racing or sculling.

So if you plan to buy home fitness equipment to improve your speed in an athletic event, you really can't go wrong.

Flexibility

Flexibility, which could be defined as the possible range of motion in a joint, or a series of joints, is, without question, one of the most important factors in a home fitness program. There are two basic types of flexibility: *static* and *dynamic.* Static flexibility is simply the measurable range of motion of a particular joint, (or series of joints). Dynamic flexibility could be thought of as the relative freedom of movement (or conversely, the stiffness) of a joint.

Flexibility is obviously important in athletics, but it is equally important in everyday life. Graceful movement depends to a large extent on flexibility. And, most importantly, a growing body of evidence indicates that maintaining good flexibility is an important factor in delaying the onset, or reducing the severity, of certain degenerative diseases. Regular stretching also prevents, or helps to relieve, some aches and pains associated both with aging and a sedentary lifestyle.

Motor coordination

Coordination of movement includes both reflex and voluntary actions of the muscles, tendons, and joints. In other words, your balance, agility, coordination, and dexterity, to a large degree, are affected by both conscious and unconscious impulses that involve the brain and nervous system.

While impulses and actions of the brain and nervous system are extremely complex, it is evident that exercise has a highly positive effect. Strength training, aerobic exercise, stretching, and an active lifestyle, helps to improve the function of the entire body. Of course, there is no substitute for improved motor coordination that results from actual practice of a sport or hobby. Skills in this area, while partly inherited, are mostly learned.

Exercise and heart rate[†]

The work load of the body is reflected by the heart rate. As work load increases, the heart rate increases accordingly, in a predictable manner. There is a point, however, at which no matter how much an individual increases the intensity of work load, the heart will not beat any faster. This point, which coincides approximately with exhaustion, is referred to as *maximal heart rate*. With age, the maximal heart rate decreases. Therefore, there is an "age adjusted maximal heart rate."

A commonly used formula for approximately predicting this maximal heart rate for both men and women is *220 minus your age*. This estimation is not precise, however, and varies to some degree among individuals.

Nonetheless, the rise in heart rate from the resting level to its maximum rate is essentially uniform, and can make an excellent monitoring device for estimating the effect of activity on the body and the heart.

With this principle in mind, you should establish a target heart rate and monitor your exercise program with the guidance of your physician. Your target heart rate is the heart rate at which you want to exercise. If you want to exercise at 50 percent of your maximal work capacity, you need to exercise at a target heart rate that is halfway between your

Exercise Target Heart Rates
(Beats per minute)

Age in Years	Percent of Maximal Work Capacity			
	40	50	60	70
20	122	135	148	161
25	120	133	146	158
30	118	130	142	154
35	116	127	139	150
40	114	125	136	147
45	112	123	133	143
50	110	120	130	140
55	108	118	127	136
60	106	115	124	133
65	104	113	121	129

Target heart rates for various ages and work capacities are listed here. Regardless of your physical condition, you should not exceed target rates listed in the far right column, which represent seventy percent of work capacity. The "talk test" is a simple rule of thumb. If you can't carry on a conversation, you're pushing too hard.

resting heart rate and your maximal heart rate.

To determine your target heart rate for fifty percent of maximal work capacity, calculate fifty percent of the difference between your adjusted maximal rate and your resting rate, then add the result to your resting heart rate. If you want to exercise at 70 percent, calculate 70 percent of the difference between your adjusted maximal rate and your resting rate, then add the result to your resting heart rate.

Since many environmental variables,

† Adapted from *Physical Fitness: How To Plan For It, Reach Your Goal, and Measure Your Progress,* by Vitamaster, Div. Allegheny Int'l. Exercise Co.

including heat, stress, noise, and anxiety, may influence an individual's resting heart rate, many people use a rate of seventy beats per minute as a standard resting heart rate.

Here's what the complete formula looks like:

Target heart rate equals

$$[(220 - Age) - 70] \times \frac{Work\ Capacity}{100} + 70$$

A table in this section uses this formula to construct target heart rates for various ages and work capacities. Age-adjusted maximal rates and the standard resting rate of seventy beats per minute were used in the computations.

Finding the best exercise level

Some conditioning effect is recognized at an exercise intensity of 40 percent of the maximal work capacity. When an individual reaches 85 percent of the maximal work capacity, there is a reduced margin of safety and an increased risk of serious rhythm disturbance. The risk is especially great if the individual has unsuspected heart disease. Most exercise prescriptions call for 50 percent of maximal work capacity, and it is recommended that the heart rate not be allowed to exceed that heart rate associated with seventy percent of the maximal work capacity.

For example, if you are forty years old and your exercise program calls for exercise at 50 percent of your maximal work capacity, then your target heart rate, as given in the table, is estimated at 125 beats per minute. You should adjust your exercise loads to maintain your heart rate around 125 beats per minute. Your heart rate should not, however, be allowed to go above 147 beats per minute, which corresponds to 70 percent of your maximal work capacity.

Knowing the heart rate provides a safety check to help prevent too much stress on the heart during an activity session. Other influences, such as environment, heat, and stress may influence heart rate response to activity. It is important that the individual not exceed his personally recommended heart rate limits, regardless of apparent work load levels. Under any circumstances, when stress symptoms occur, or heart rate limits are reached, you should limit your activity.

It also is important to recognize the potential hazards of excessive physical activity, especially exercise rates. Most exercise prescriptions call for 50 percent of maximal work capacity. Above 60 percent, physical and chemical stresses, which may become hazardous, begin in the body. Above 85 percent, there is a very significant risk of heart rhythm disturbance, or other complications, particularly in the person with heart disease.

Physical educators use the "talk test" as an indicator of work load. At about 60 percent of maximal work capacity, mouth breathing begins. At 70 percent, communication is limited, and, at 85 percent, the participant is not interested in talking at all. For safety, therefore, the individual should "keep his (or her) reserve" and remain able to carry on a conversation at all times. The level of exercise should be sufficiently vigorous to provide physical conditioning, but not so strenuous as to be harmful.

Remember, remain comfortable while exercising! Don't push yourself to the point of symptoms! For safety, you should always be able to carry on a conversation.

Fitness planning

Your program of physical activities should be planned and gradual, varied and safe. Understanding the principles of physical activity, aided by the use of exercise equipment, should help you become healthier, happier, and more fit through a safe and planned program.

The principle factors of the exercise program, whether your goal is for weight control, to improve the cardiorespiratory system, or for general conditioning, are the same: the work load during exercise; the duration of the exercise session; and the frequency of exercise sessions. Careful attention to the heart rate, and to any unusual symptoms that may arise, are the keys to safety.

The objective of your exercise program is to progress gradually over a period of weeks up to the point at which you are able to exercise for up to twenty minutes each session, monitoring your heart rate so that you do not exceed 70 percent of maximal work capacity. You should exercise three to five times each week. The duration of each exercise session after you are in shape should be such that the total time of exercise each week maintains your acquired conditioning level. Maintenance usually requires at least three twenty-minute sessions per week.

A "warm-up" of five to ten minutes is important to protect muscles and prepare the cardiorespiratory system for exercise. Flexing and extending your muscles will help. After exercise, remember that a five to ten minute "cool-down," consisting of walking or slow pedaling on an exercise cycle, is extremely important to return the cardiovascular system to a lower level of function. Heart rhythm disturbances may occur during the immediate post-exercise period; the "cool-down" session is important to protect against this.

In order to condition the cardiorespiratory system, a schedule such as that shown on the table in this section, is suggested to bring yourself gradually into condition.

The target heart rate should be selected on the basis of your physical fitness status classifications and a physician's advice and clearance. An intensity of 40 percent of the maximal work capacity is desired for some conditioning effect. Most initial exercise prescriptions call for 50 percent of maximal capacity. Above 60 percent, hazardous physical and chemical stresses may begin in the body. Above 85 percent, there is a very

Sample Cardiorespiratory Conditioning Program

Time/Session (minutes)						
Exercise Week	Warm-up	Target Heart Rate	Cool-down	Total Time	Frequency Sessions/ Wk	Exercise Time/Wk
1 & 2	3	3	4	10	5	50
3 & 4	4	4	4	12	5	60
5 & 6	4	6	5	15	5	75
7 & 8	5	8	5	18	5	90
9 & 10	5	10	5	20	5	100
11 & 12	6	12	6	24	5	120

Note: Target heart rate is usually expressed as that heart rate associated with fifty percent of maximal work capacity. The heart rate should not be allowed to exceed the rate associated with seventy percent of maximal work capacity. The amount of elapsed time during which the target heart rate is sustained is the time during which the heart rate exceeds the rate associated with forty percent of maximal work capacity.

significant risk of heart rhythm disturbances, or other complications. Therefore, it is recommended that the heart rate not be allowed to exceed 70 percent of the maximal work capacity.

For example, in the case of a forty-year-old whose exercise program calls for exercise at 50 percent of the maximal work capacity, and who has progressed to the third week of the cardiorespiratory conditioning program, the exercise session as given in the table would call for the following sequence:

■ 1. Warm up on an exercise cycle (rowing machine, treadmill, etc.) for approximately four minutes.
■ 2. Increase the work load on the cycle (or other fitness machine) to elevate the heart rate to that level associated with more than 40 percent of the maximal work capacity or, as given in the table, as 114 beats per minute.
■ 3. As the heart rate approaches the heart rate associated with 50 percent of the maximal work capacity, or 125 beats per minute, adjust the load level to maintain this heart rate.
■ 4. The heart rate should never be allowed to reach 147 beats per minute, which corresponds to 70 percent of the maximal work capacity.
■ 5. According to the table, the individual should exercise with the heart rate above 114 beats per minute for four minutes.
■ 6. After four minutes, the load should be reduced to a no-load condition, and exercise continued for a cool-down period of four or more minutes.

Each session should follow the same general sequence specified in the table. However, as you progress through the weeks, the conditioning effect will enable you to maintain the heart rate at target levels for longer periods of time, or to overcome higher loads on the exercise cycle (or other piece of equipment) to achieve the target heart rate. This represents improvement of functional capacity, or fitness.

If you have reached your weight goal, or if your cardiorespiratory system is in such good condition that you are able to function within your target heart rate zone without any problems, you will still have to exercise regularly if you do not want to lose the benefits for which you have worked so hard. If you stop your program, most of what you have worked for will be lost in approximately three to six weeks.

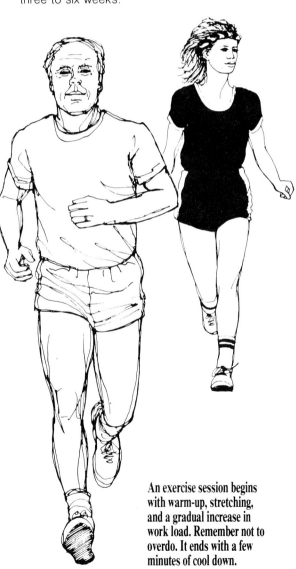

An exercise session begins with warm-up, stretching, and a gradual increase in work load. Remember not to overdo. It ends with a few minutes of cool down.

Warm-ups

These prepare the body for more vigorous exercise and should be done with enough energy to increase the body's central temperature, usually recognized by the appearance of sweating. This increases the body's efficiency by making the muscles more fluid and shortening reflex times. The gentle stretching prepares ligaments for further stretching-with less danger of being sprained-and stimulates the tonic relfexes* of muscles to help protect them from strain. Since the heart rate is increased, the heart will reach its rate of maximum efficiency more quickly.

These exercises don't have to follow a formed sequence. All body areas that will be involved in the more vigorous exercises to follow should be included in the warm-ups, which should take three to five minutes.

*Reflexes that maintain posture

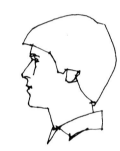

1. Head and neck
   a. Head flexion and extension
   b. Head rotation in alternate direction (chin held level)

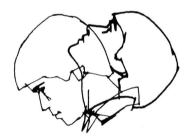

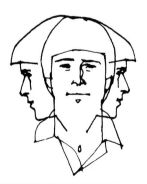

Source: American Medical Association

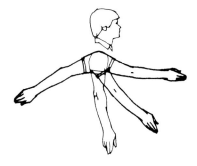

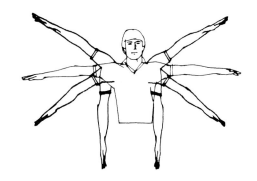

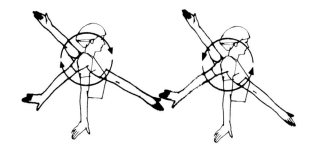

2. Upper extremities

   a. Arm swings-forward, backward and
      sideward

   b. Arm circles, forward and backward

   c. Overhead reach, alternate arms

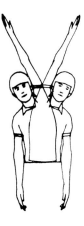

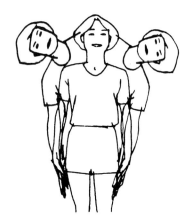

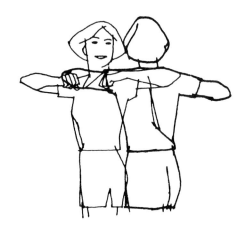

3. Trunk
    a. Sideward trunk bends, both sides
    b. Trunk twist (shoulder level)
    c. Knee to chest pressor (standing or with
       elbow support in supine position)

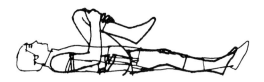

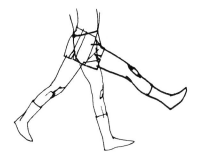

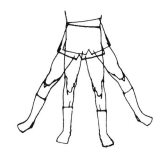

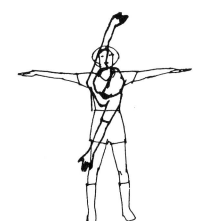

4. Lower extremities
  a. Alternate leg raising-forward, backward and
     sideward (standing or lying on side)
  b. Windmill
  c. Toe-touching

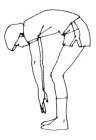

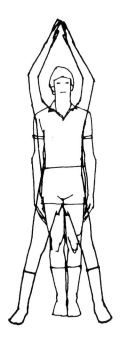

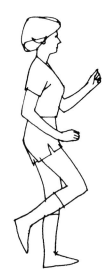

5. Cardiopulmonary

a. Jumping jacks
b. Run-walk in place
c. Hop five left, five right

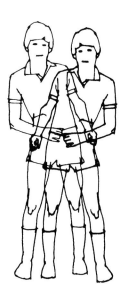

Vigorous activities

One or more of the activities listed in the chart below should be performed for twenty or more minutes. The same activities can be performed each session, or the activities can be varied from session to session.

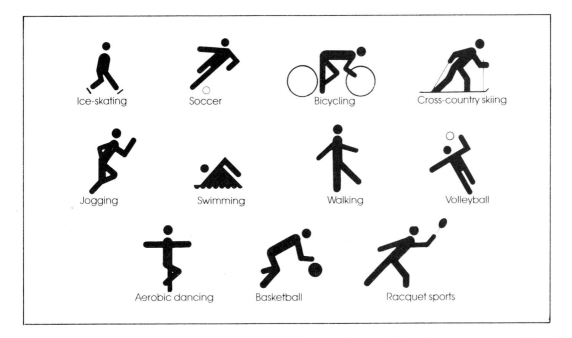

Cooling down

1. Walk about breathing deeply.
2. A period of relaxation prior to resuming normal activities.
3. It is not advisable to abruptly alter body temperature by:
   - a. shower
   - b. sauna
   - c. whirlpool
   - d. swimming pool
   - e. steam bath

(These activities can be undertaken after a cool-down period.)

Exercise Diary

Make photocopies of these pages. Take the diary to your workout. On a scale of one to five, record pre-exercise stress level (one being minimal stress, five being highly stressed). Describe your exercise activity, location, time of day, and length of workout. Record pre-exercise heart-rate, range of heart-rate during exercise, and post-exercise recovery heart rate (taken one minute following exercise). On a scale from one to five, record your attitude regarding outcome of workout (one being poor, five being great).

DATE: WEIGHT: HOURS OF SLEEP NIGHT BEFORE:

	AEROBIC	STRENGTH	FLEXIBILITY
PRE-EXERCISE STRESS LEVEL			
DESCRIPTION and LOCATION of ACTIVITY			
TIME of DAY			
LENGTH of WORKOUT			
HEART RATES PRE DURING POST			
POST-EXERCISE ATTITUDE			

Source: Charts and advice courtesy of Campbell's Institute for Health and Fitness, Turnaround Leaders Workshop. For more information, write to Campbell's Institute for Health and Fitness, Camden, New Jersey 08101.

DATE:	WEIGHT:		HOURS OF SLEEP NIGHT BEFORE:
	AEROBIC	STRENGTH	FLEXIBILITY
PRE-EXERCISE STRESS LEVEL			
DESCRIPTION and LOCATION of ACTIVITY			
TIME of DAY			
LENGTH of WORKOUT			
HEART RATES PRE DURING POST			
POST-EXERCISE ATTITUDE			

DATE:	WEIGHT:		HOURS OF SLEEP NIGHT BEFORE:
	AEROBIC	STRENGTH	FLEXIBILITY
PRE-EXERCISE STRESS LEVEL			
DESCRIPTION and LOCATION of ACTIVITY			
TIME of DAY			
LENGTH of WORKOUT			
HEART RATES PRE DURING POST			
POST-EXERCISE ATTITUDE			

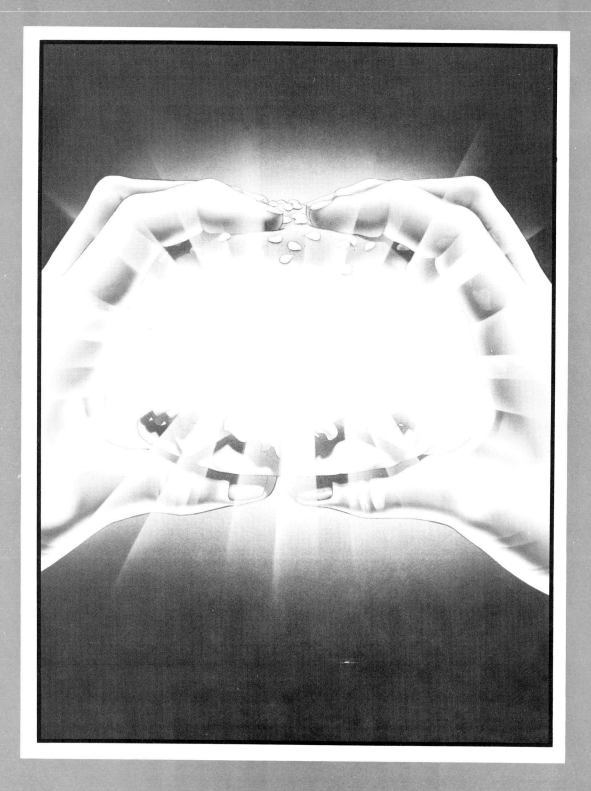

Eating right

The adult diet

During the long and active period of adulthood, people experiment with many new foods and combinations of foods. Although there is no single right way of eating, the foods selected should add up to a diet that provides all the nutrients needed for good health.

The most common nutrition problem of adults in the United States is obesity. Another common problem is iron deficiency in women of childbearing age. Protein and vitamin deficiencies are uncommon, and when they do occur, they are usually secondary to other problems, such as alcoholism, other serious or chronic illness, a very unusual diet, or inadequate income.

Some people fall into the habit of taking multi-vitamin supplements for "insurance" and then don't think much about the foods they eat. Others have the conviction that their health depends on an array of supplements, such as vitamins, minerals, protein, lecithin, and so on. With the thousands of supplements on the market today, however, it is far more difficult to make safe and rational decisions about supplements than it is to plan an adequate diet of ordinary foods.

Weight control

If you plan on losing some weight, your diet should be as normal as possible. Foods should be chosen from each of the four groups (see chart on page 175), but the choices can be modified somewhat to reduce total calories. This means using low-fat or nonfat dairy products instead of whole milk, leaner cuts and smaller servings of meats, the minimum number of recommended servings of breads and cereals, and fruits and vegetables without syrups and sauces. It does *not* mean eliminating any of these important food groups.

In order to prevent a gradual weight gain over the years, individuals in their twenties should take a realistic look at their diet and exercise patterns. After high school or college days are over, there may be fewer athletic events, dances, and other activities to justify a high-calorie intake.

There is no diet that can bring about physical fitness in a person who is not physically active. For good health throughout adulthood, the best approach is through weight control, adequate diet, and regular exercise.

Exercise and weight control

The key to effective weight control is to balance calorie intake with energy output. When calories consumed exceed those required to meet the body's needs, the excess will be stored as fat unless physical activity is increased proportionately. This is true for both sexes at all ages.

In their attempts to lose excess fat and prevent unwanted weight gains, many people concentrate on counting food calories and neglect the role of exercise in increasing energy output. Studies comparing food intake and activity patterns of overweight people with those of people with normal weight indicate that lack of exercise is more often the cause of overweight than overeating. In all age levels studied, overweight people did not consume more calories than their normal-weight age mates, but they led much more sedentary lives. This lack of exercise is to some extent a by-product of increasing urban living, greater reliance on automobiles and greater use of labor-saving devices.

It takes effort and willpower to counter these trends by creating opportunities for regular vigorous exercise. Although daily weight loss may be small, continuation of your exercise program can lead to loss of four to six pounds in a month and fifty to sixty pounds in a year, provided that food consumption remains the same. The reverse is also true. Just one extra slice of buttered toast a day, or one soft drink, or any other food item that contains about 100 calories, can add up to ten extra pounds in a year if you don't increase your physical activity at the same time.

The notion that exercise must be exhausting to produce dividends is misleading. Although it takes an hour's jogging to use up 600 calories, you don't have to do it all in one stretch; a half hour uses up 300 calories.

Energy expended is also affected by body weight. In activities where a person has to move his own weight, energy output is increased for the heavier person and decreased for the lighter. The more weight you need to lose, the more you will benefit from moderate exercise.

It has been suggested that appetite will increase as exercise increases, so that the balance between energy intake and output will not change. In fact, those who exercise more do not always eat more, and with regular programs of vigorous exercise, appetite may decrease as energy output increases.

A lean person in good condition may eat more following increased activity, but his exercise will burn up the extra calories he consumes. The overweight person often doesn't react the same way to exercise. Because he has large stores of fat, moderate exercise often does not stimulate his appetite.

Laboratory tests on experimental animals have shown the difference in response to exercise in fat and lean people. In one experiment, animals exercised vigorously over longer periods ate more, but the extra activity kept their weights constant. In other experiments, when the animals' activity was decreased, they continued to eat the same amount of food and gained weight.

Similarly, a study of overweight adults showed that the start of their obesity corresponded with their decline in activity.

Daily Food Guide

The recommended servings of foods from each group are the minimum servings needed each day for an adult. The minimum servings listed will provide about 1,300 calories, and from eight to 120 percent of the Recommended Daily Allowance (RDA) of nutrients.

The Daily Food Guide is only the foundation upon which a good diet is built. Individuals can fully meet their calorie and nutrient needs by having more and larger servings of foods from the basic diet and by adding other foods that are called "extras."

Milk Group
(includes milk or yogurt)   2 cups or more

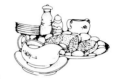

Meat Group
(includes meat, fish, poultry, eggs)

2 servings or more

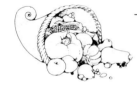

Vegetable and Fruit Group

A: Vitamin-C rich: Citrus fruits and   1 serving
juices, such as cantaloupe, fresh
strawberries, broccoli, tomatoes

B: For vitamin-A: Carrots, broccoli,   1 serving
cooked greens and dark salad greens,
sweet potatoes, apricots, winter
squash

C: Potatoes, other vegetables and   2 servings
fruits

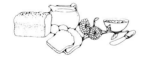

Bread-Cereal Group

Whole grain and enriched: cereals,   4 servings
breads, rice, macaroni, noodles, spa-
ghetti

Extras
Butter, margarine,
salad oils (in tablespoons)   Sugars, syrups,   Use in moderation
honey and other sweets
2-3 servings

Many foods can be substituted for those listed in the Daily Food Guide. For example, cheese and ice cream can replace part of the milk requirement. One cup of milk is equal to about one and one-fourth ounces of either cottage cheese or ice cream. It also is important to drink enough fluids-at least four to five cups a day.

A serving of meat, fish, poultry, or eggs can be alternated with cheese, dried beans, peas or lentils, or peanut butter. About three ounces of meat comprise and adult-size serving.

Women should be careful to eat plenty of iron-rich foods, especially during pregnancy, because females are prone to iron deficiency. Iron-rich foods include liver, heart, lean meat, shellfish, egg yolks, legumes, green leafy vegetables, and whole-grain or enriched breads and cereal products.

"Extras" include not only fats and sugars, but also alcohol, cookies, cakes, pastries, chips and dips, candy and other unclassified items. These foods should be minor rather than major items in the diet.

Source: American Medical Association

This is a common observation. When people finish school and go to work (especially if the job is a sedentary one), they tend to exercise less, but through habit eat as much as ever. And before long, they are overweight.

Dieting

If weight control can be achieved either through dieting or exercise, wouldn't it be easier to concentrate on dieting and not worry about exercise?

A sensible diet-one that includes foods in moderate amounts from the basic food groups-may help you to lose weight without giving up good nutrition. But no diet lasts forever. Once you've reached a desirable weight, you'll tend to return to your normal eating habits with an increased caloric intake. Unless you increase your physical activity at this point, your weight loss will not be maintained.

What about "crash" or very restricted diets? Remarkable claims have been made for

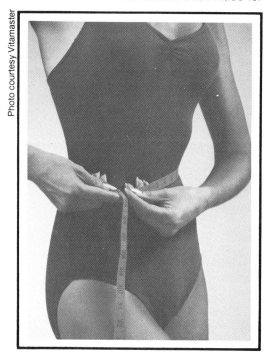

Photo courtesy Vitamaster

a variety of these.

Some crash diets do achieve noticeable weight loss in a short time, and such a loss is quickly restored when regular eating habits are resumed. Body fat, on the other hand, is lost very slowly. This is why some dieters become discouraged quickly and conclude that losing weight for them is impossible. Extreme calorie reduction over extended periods, unless under medical supervision, may create nutritional problems. Recent studies have shown that weight reduction through near starvation may be at the expense of valuable body tissues rather than reduction of fat.

No room for compromise

If you want to lose weight, exercise is of great importance. But remember, increasing your level of physical activity doesn't give you a license also to increase your diet! Step up the exercise, but keep your diet well-balanced with about the same caloric intake-or a little less-for best long-term results.

Remember also that the exercises you choose should be vigorous enough to use up the required number of calories and that they should be done on a regular basis.

You may follow your new program for several days and find no difference on the bathroom scale. Adjustments in metabolism take place, and it may be some time before any weight loss can be seen. In exercising regularly, some flabby tissue is changed to muscle tissue that may weigh as much, but takes up less space. Thus, a trimmer figure results, even though weight may not drop markedly.

Supplements

Supplements are needed only when you are unable or unwilling to consume an adequate diet. Healthy people rarely require supplements. It is healthier, cheaper, and easier to eat a balanced diet than to pop

Suggested weights for heights

You can probably tell whether you have a weight problem and how serious it is simply by looking in a mirror, or referring to a height/weight table. The height/weight table has the advantage of being objective and impersonal. What it tells you about your weight may be more reliable than your own impression, or that of your friends and relatives. Still, the table has its limitations. Both underweight and overweight people may try to use the table in such a way as to justify their weights.

In order to estimate your ideal weight, you must compare your own body build to that of an imaginary "average" person of your height. Persons with a large build (wide shoulders and hips, large wrists and ankles) can estimate their best weight to be somewhere between the "average" and "high" figures on the table. Those with small builds (narrow shoulders and hips, small wrists and ankles) probably should weigh no more than the average and no less than the figure in the "low" column. Most people, however, are of medium build and can use the column for average weights.

Sedentary people may weigh just what the table suggests, yet have too much fat in relation to lean tissue to be considered physically fit. Remember, the table has its limitations.

Height (without shoes) Feet Inches	Weight (without clothing) Pounds		
● Men	Low	Average	High
5'3"	118	129	141
5'4"	122	133	145
5'5"	126	137	149
5'6"	130	142	155
5'7"	134	147	161
5'8"	139	151	166
5'9"	143	155	170
5'10"	147	159	174
5'11"	150	163	178
6'	154	167	183
6'1"	158	171	188
6'2"	162	175	192
6'3"	165	178	195
● Women			
5'	100	109	118
5'1"	104	112	121
5'2"	107	115	125
5'3"	110	118	128
5'4"	113	122	132
5'5"	116	125	135
5'6"	120	129	139
5'7"	123	132	142
5'8"	126	136	146
5'9"	130	140	151
5'10"	133	144	156
5'11"	137	148	161
6'	141	152	166

Source: U.S. Dept. of Agriculture (for height/weight figures). "The Healthy Approach to Slimming," copyright 1984, American Medical Association. Used with permission.

vitamin and mineral pills.

Of course, there are exceptions. Some women may require additional iron in their diets, especially during menstruation or pregnancy. In addition, alcoholics, habitual dieters, and elderly people frequently have inadequate diets. While vitamin and mineral supplements are recommended as short-term solutions to inadequate diets in these cases, the recommended long-term solution is to improve the diet.

If you feel you absolutely must supplement your diet with vitamins and minerals, look for a supplement that contains vitamin and mineral levels that fall within the Recommended Dietary Allowances approved by the United States Food and Drug Administration (FDA). These supplements provide all the vitamins and minerals needed by just about anybody.

High-potency supplements

There is considerable controversy over the use of high-potency supplements by athletes and health food enthusiasts. The American Medical Association recommends avoiding the use of high-potency supplements unless they are prescribed by a doctor. These are supplements that are frequently sold through the mail or over-the-counter through various retail outlets.

Many physicians and pharmacists believe that these mega-dose supplements provide little or no benefits other than enriching the vitamin content of the buyer's urine. This is because vitamins, by nature, are needed in very small amounts by the body. At excessive levels, the water soluble ones such as Vitamin C and the B-complex vitamins are excreted.

But that's not all. Vitamins stop acting like vitamins at high dosages; their activity changes to drug-like action.

The problem with mineral supplements is that a large dose of one type can interfere with the body's use of another. Doctors recommend the use of mineral supplements, such as iron, only when there is evidence of deficiency or increased need.

A reasonable supplement contains 50 to 150 percent of the United States Recommended Daily Amounts (RDA) for vitamins and minerals. Exceptions are vitamins A and D, which should not exceed 100 percent because they are non-water-soluble and accumulate in body fat over long periods of time.

For most of us, it is a lot easier and more sensible to eat a balanced diet.

Sodium

Sodium is a mineral that combines easily with other chemical elements. It occurs naturally in many foods and is added to many others. The most typical sodium compounds in foods include salt, baking soda, and baking powder. Sodium is also found in many preservatives, flavorings, and sweeteners.

Small quantities of sodium are necessary to the normal function of the heart and other muscles. For many people, however, dietary intake of sodium far exceeds the amount needed for good health. Scientists have established a relationship between sodium intake and the potential for development or control of high blood pressure. More than nineteen million people in the United States are hypertensive, and another eighteen million are borderline hypertensive.

Fortunately, most people probably are not predisposed to developing hypertension. But for those at risk, doctors frequently prescribe low-sodium diets.

The Food and Nutrition Board of the National Academy of Sciences has established 1,100 to 3,300 milligrams of sodium a day as a ''safe and adequate'' range of intake.

U.S Recommended Daily Allowances (U.S. RDA)

(For use in nutrition labeling of foods, including dietary supplements of vitamins and minerals)

	Adults and Children Over 4 years	Pregnant or Breast-feeding Women
Vitamin A, I.U.	5,000	8,000
Vitamin C, mg	60	60
Vitamin D, I.U.	400	400
Vitamin E, I.U.	30	30
Thiamin, mg	1.5	1.7
Riboflavin, mg	1.7	2.0
Niacin, mg	20	20
Vitamin B_6, mg	2.0	2.5
Vitamin B_{12}, mcg	6	8
Folic acid, mg	0.4	0.8
Biotin, mg*	0.3	0.3
Pantothenic acid, mg*	10	10
Calcium, g	1.0	1.3
Phosphorus, g	1.0	1.3
Iron, mg	18	18
Zinc, mg	15	15
Magnesium, mg	400	450
Copper, mg*	2.0	2.0
Iodine, mcg	150	150
Protein, g**	65	65

*Recommended Dietary Allowances for these nutrients have not been established by the Food and Nutrition Board, National Academy of Sciences—National Research Council.

**If protein efficiency ratio is equal to or better than that of casein, U.S. RDA is 45 grams for adults and pregnant or lactating women, 20 grams for children under four years of age, and 18 grams for infants.

Sources: Food and Nutrition Board, National Academy of Sciences-National Research Council.

Daily food diary

Day: Date:

Time	Where	Associated activity	"Slowing"	Impor-tant	Food and amount	Calories
6-11 am						
11-4 pm						
4-9 pm						
9 pm-6 am						
					Total	

Daily food diary

Instructions for using the Food Diary

Carry the Diary with you and complete it right after eating. Note the time when you started eating. Note where you were eating. Note what you were doing while eating (e.g. reading, cooking, watching television, etc.). Place a check in the "Slowing" column if you practiced eating more slowly. Place a check in the "Importance" column if you really felt this meal or snack was important to you. Fill in the food and amount. Look up and enter the number of calories in each food (there are many calorie guides available, but choose a respected source). At the end of the week, complete the "Weekly Summary." Try to remember the physical activities you did during the week.

Weekly food diary

In filling in the "Weekly Summary," enter your daily intake of calories and compute the weekly average. Do the same for meals and snacks. Count the number of times you practiced "slowing." Count the number of times each day you ate but didn't consider the eating important. Note any special efforts at increasing physical activity and calories expended in that activity. During the next week, see if you can't improve: fewer calories, remember trade-offs, more slowing, and try to eliminate unimportant eating.

	Calories	Meals	Snacks	How many times did you practice Slowing?	How many times did you consider Meals or Snacks Important?	Activity	Calories Expended in Activity
Mon.							
Tues.							
Wed.							
Thurs.							
Fri.							
Sat.							
Sun.							
Total							
Daily average							

Source: Charts and advice courtesy of Campbell's Institute for Health and Fitness, Turnaround Leaders Kit. For more information, write to Campbell's Institute for Health and Fitness, Camden, New Jersey 08101.

Index

Index

By topic